July 9/ 1999

SPINAL MANIPULATION

Spinal Manipulation

J. F. Bourdillon FRCS FRCS (C)

Past President, North American Academy of
Manipulative Medicine
Formerly Consultant Orthopaedic Surgeon to the
Gloucestershire Royal Hospital
Associate Clinical Professor (Orthopaedic Surgery)
College of Osteopathic Medicine, Michigan State University

E. A. Day MD FRCP (C)

Specialist in Physical Medicine and Rehabilitation, Ottawa

Fourth Edition

William Heinemann Medical Books
London

Appleton
&Lange
Norwalk, Connecticut / Los Altos, California

William Heinemann Medical Books,
22 Bedford Square,
London WC1B 3HH

ISBN 0–433–03633–8 (UK)
ISBN 0–8385–8642–2 (USA)

First published 1970
Second Edition 1973
Revised reprint 1975
Third Edition 1982
Fourth Edition 1987

US edition

Distributed in Continental North America, Hawaii,
Puerto Rico and Canada by Appleton & Lange.

Filmset and printed in Great Britain by
BAS Printers Limited, Over Wallop, Hampshire

Contents

Preface to the First Edition

So many people have helped me in my efforts to produce this book that it would be impossible to mention them all.

I must gratefully acknowledge the permission given by the British Medical Journal for the extracts from a 1910 Editorial; from H. K. Lewis & Company Limited to quote from Timbrell Fisher's Treatment by Manipulation; from the J. B. Lippincott Company for permission to quote from an article by Dr Horace Gray in the International Clinics, and from the Editors of Brain and the Anatomical Record for permission to reproduce the dermatome charts in the papers by Sir Henry Head and by Drs Keegan and Garrett respectively.

It is invidious to thank individuals but I must express my gratitude for the cheerful and untiring help which I have received from the British Columbia Medical Library Service and from the Staff of the Records Department of the Gloucestershire Royal Hospital.

I cannot leave out my secretary who has typed, typed and retyped every word that is here written, nor indeed, my wife, who has in turn typed, criticised, encouraged and proof read. Finally, it would be very discourteous not to mention both my long suffering model and her husband who took the photographs.

I have endeavoured to shed light on the mystery that surrounds manipulation, to explain how to do it in terms that I hope will be easy enough to understand, to produce a working hypothesis as a basis for argument and a guide for research, and to show some of the reasons why I believe that it is essential that Medicine should incorporate this teaching into its structure.

Vancouver, B.C.   J.F.B.
1970

Preface to the Fourth Edition

In the Fourth Edition the author of the previous editions has been joined by Dr Edward A. Day, MD, FRCP (Canada) a graduate of Dalhousie University in Halifax, Nova Scotia. Dr Day is a specialist in Physical Medicine and Rehabilitation and brings the outlook of a different specialty to the opinions expressed. He also is a practitioner of the type of manipulative procedures described in this book.

In this edition the chapters on examination and treatment have been largely rewritten and expanded. The chapter on anatomy has been expanded to include the areas needed for the new treatment text. The thoracic cage has been dealt with as a separate chapter with a much more inclusive description of methods of diagnosing and treating rib dysfunctions. An endeavour has been made to present at least the method of making a diagnosis and a means of treating all except the rarest of the dysfunctions of the axial skeleton, pelvis and ribs. It is recognised that there are many techniques for treatment which are not included, indeed there are nearly as many techniques as there are manipulators!

Many of the illustrations are new and of these the majority will be seen to be of male models. In spite of this, in the interest of clarity, the notation used in earlier editions has been retained. The operator is designated by the male gender and the patient by the female. Our thanks are due in particular to the three new models, to those who took the photographs and those who helped to lessen the number of mistakes, including the publishers and their most assiduous freelance editor, Jane Smith.

Other sections of the book have also been altered. The appendix has been omitted and new chapters added on clinical observations and the validation of manipulation.

It is perhaps unexpected to find a man trained as an orthodox orthopaedic surgeon (JFB) writing as a protagonist of manipulative therapy of the kind described in this book, and a brief explanation is appropriate. My early interest in the subject was stimulated by a series of coincidences which led to an appreciation of its importance in spite of the early 'brainwashing' to which I was subjected.

While still a preclinical student I sustained a severe strain of my lumbar spine as a result of a motorcycle accident, and I continued to suffer symptoms from this almost continuously for a number of years and at intervals ever since. I was treated initially, first by one and then by a second very well-known orthopaedic surgeon, but the treatments which I received had no effect whatever on the condition other than to give me temporary relief at the time of administration of heat and massage. I well remember the black looks I used to get from the ward sister on teaching rounds in St Thomas' Hospital in the days when Dame Lloyd Still was matron. When I stood for more than 10 minutes at a time my back began to ache so badly that I found it necessary to rest my buttocks on some sort of support and the neighbouring bed was by far the easiest. This disarranged the bed cover and was the cause of the sister's displeasure.

During my war service with the Royal Air Force, I was well grounded in the treatment of acute trauma but the chronic back condition was relatively rare and my introduction to these in quantity came after my return as senior registrar to St Thomas' Hospital, where I quickly learned the then new operation of removal of the protruded intervertebral disc. At first it seemed that this might be the answer to the problem, but disillusionment very quickly followed in the wake of negative exploration and unsatisfactory postoperative results. Like many others, I had originally been taught that manipulation under general anaesthetic of the spine of a patient with backache was dangerous and the more so if there was coexistent sciatica. In my case the teaching resulted from the unfortunate experience of two of my tutors, in which the manipulation under anaesthetic of the spine of a doctor's wife produced a permanent cauda equina paralysis.

I completed my registrar training in Cambridge, where I learned from R. W. Butler his technique of manipulating spines under general anaesthetic with good results and without any accidents. Working for him I naturally observed and followed his techniques, often with a very satisfactory measure of success. One of the basic points that he taught was a strict avoidance of forced flexion of the spine. The manipulation consisted of traction, rotation and extension only.

I had the good fortune to be called to see a woman with a recurrence of old back trouble. She described how her general practitioner relieved her by a simple manipulation and explained to me how he did it. The movement was similar to one which I had been using under anaesthesia but was accomplished easily and almost without pain. She obtained immediate relief and only required one treatment. Later I discovered the need of repeated treatment in many cases in order to give lasting relief.

By this time I was using techniques similar to those used by Butler but without anaesthesia because I found it to be unnecessary and because of the need for repeated treatment. I have now come to believe that the use of anaesthesia is a great mistake except for very exceptional circumstances. The intense muscle spasm over destructive lesions is a very valuable ally because it prevents damage being done even if one should misdiagnose such a lesion in the early stages and manipulate it. Anaesthesia will, of course, diminish or even abolish the muscle spasm.

When I first started manipulating spines I was doing it solely for problems in the back itself. I quickly began to find that I was relieving pain in the arms or legs at the same time, even when the symptomatology had not been such as to make me feel that the pain was a referred one. At that time I still believed in the theory that pressure on nerves was the chief cause of referred pain. My continuing experience led me to have serious doubts and at least tended to make me think.

My interest in the other schools of manipulative therapy was stimulated by a number of patients whose backs I had manipulated without success, who were kind enough to let me know that subsequent visits to non-medically qualified manipulators had given satisfactory relief. This naturally made me wish to study the methods used by these practitioners. The rules of the profession made this somewhat difficult until by chance I met the late Dr Donald Turner, then a general practitioner in Folkestone, who himself had learnt the techniques after being relieved of a severe sciatica by an osteopath. He was kind enough to teach me what he knew and from this and from other medical manipulators I developed the system which I have used for many years and which I have tried to describe under the heading of semispecific (or 'simpler') treatment. I have subsequently learned the more specific methods, chiefly from members of the osteopathic profession, some of whose work is referred to in the references in Chapter 3.

Lantzville, B.C.   J.F.B.
1987

Chapter 1

Introduction

The art of manipulation of the spine is a very old one. It has been practised since prehistoric times and was known to Hippocrates and to the physicians of ancient Rome.

Bone setters have existed for as long as there are records, and in many countries, including England, they still exist. In the library of the Royal College of Surgeons in London is a book dated 1656 which is a revision by one Robert Turner of a work by an Augustinian monk, Friar Moulton, entitled *The Compleat Bone Setter*.

One of the authors (EAD) has had the experience of using manipulative methods on patients from as diverse places as Mexico and Iran only to have the patient say that he had someone in the village who did that too!

In 1745 the surgeons eventually separated from the old City of London Company of Barbers and Surgeons of London and formed a new company which, in the early nineteenth century, became the Royal College of Surgeons of England.

Prior to this time it is probable that the bone setters were regarded as the orthopaedic surgeons of their day, but for reasons that are unknown they became less and less respected as the art of medicine and surgery gradually became transformed into a science.

The art of bone setting appears often to have been passed from father to son, and there is some evidence to suggest that an hereditary trait is of some value. Certainly it is accepted that some learn the art of manipulation much more easily than others. The art was not at any time supported by adequate scientific investigation, but experience with patients previously handled by bone setters shows that these practitioners are sometimes surprisingly skilful. Unfortunately their explanation to their clients of what they do is often quite unacceptable to the medical profession and reflects their almost total lack of knowledge of anatomy, physiology or pathology.

The advent of routine radiography, the research into the anatomy of the intervertebral joint and of the disc, and operative findings have conclusively shown that there is not 'a little bone out of place'. The orthodox medical profession has, therefore, found itself unable to accept the manipulators' claims. Unfortunately, the rejection of these claims has provided the profession with a most convenient cloak behind which to hide its refusal to acknowledge the manipulators' success and its dislike of anything new and strange. This, however, is a poor excuse for failure to investigate, test and research into the treatment which these practitioners use, even if it were less successful than it is known to be.

It is easy in this modern day to forget that only a few generations ago medicine was an art and the large majority of medical and surgical treatments were based on the results of practical experience rather than on firm scientific foundation. There are still many procedures being carried out without ever having been subjected to scientific scrutiny. Carotid endarterectomy appears to be an example: in an article in the Canadian journal *The Medical Post*, dated February 4th 1986, it was announced that a multicentre trial had been started in the USA to assess the risks and benefits of this 'unproven multi-billion-dollar industry'.

The reasons for the neglect of research into the art of manipulation are manifold, but the results of this neglect are potentially serious to the profession. It has already resulted in the development of two schools of manipulative treatment separate from the profession as well as in the continued prosperity of a multitude of irregular practitioners styling themselves under a variety of names.

The celebrated John Hunter is quoted by Timbrell Fisher[1] as having said: 'Nothing can promote contracture of a joint so much as motion before the disease is removed . . . When all inflammation has gone off and healing has begun, a little motion frequently repeated is necessary to prevent healing taking place with the parts fixed in one position.' This, unfortunately, was interpreted by Hunter's successors in such a way that they felt justified in allowing adhesions to form in a joint and relying on their ability afterwards to mobilise them.

This treatment is still accepted as being of the greatest value in infective arthritis. Unfortunately, the concept was extended to joints stiffened by injury and it is now well known that in such patients early movement of the injured joint is a much more reliable method of restoring function.

It must be remembered that, at that time, there were no x-rays, tuberculosis was common in England, and diagnosis presented serious difficulties. The standard of orthodox treatment for joint disease was far from satisfactory, many ending up with a joint excision or amputation. At the same time the fear of litigation against bone setters was almost non-existent and there can be no doubt that patients were injured by forcible manipulation of infected joints.

The famous British surgeon Sir James Paget was one of the few of his day who appreciated the value of manipulative therapy and in his lecture published in the *British Medical Journal*[2] he gave the following advice: 'Learn then, to imitate what is good and avoid what is bad in the practice of bone setters . . . too long rest is, I believe, by far the most frequent cause of delayed recovery after injuries of joints and not only to injured joints, but to those that are kept at rest because parts near them have been injured.'

The medical profession of the time paid little heed to Paget's advice. Hugh Owen Thomas used to teach that an overdose of rest was impossible, an idea that appears to have taken root at a time when he had a bitter quarrel with his father who, like his grandfather, was a bone setter. He is quoted by Timbrell Fisher[1] as having written a letter in reply to Paget's lecture in which he said: 'For many years after the commencement of my experience in surgery I had the opportunity of observing the practice of those who had acquired a good reputation for skill as successful manipulators . . . I cannot find suitable cases on which I would perform the deception known as passive motion.'

Later, however, his own suffering led Thomas to visit one of the most celebrated bone setters of the nineteenth century and the following passage in another letter, quoted by Timbrell Fisher,[1] reflects the change of heart produced by personal experience.

> In my own case, after submitting to Mr. Hutton's manipulation, I was instantly relieved of that pain, tension and coldness in the joint that I had suffered for six years, and was able to walk . . . Professional men accounted for the manifest change in my condition on one hypothesis and another, whilst all affected to smile at my ignorance and delusion . . . I had been lame and in pain and could now walk and was at ease . . . and had the whole College of Surgeons clearly demonstrated to their entire satisfaction that I could not possibly have been benefited by Mr. Hutton's treatment, my opinion would not have been in the smallest degree shaken by it.

One of the difficulties arises from the fact that the symptoms produced by a spinal joint derangement can be surprisingly diverse and are often manifest at a distance from the spine rather than in the spine itself. Another arises from the anatomy, the spinal joint being situated deep beneath powerful muscles so that it is only indirectly available to the examining finger. A possible third is that the art of successful spinal manipulation comes much more easily to some people than to others. It is a skill which comes with training and perseverance but, as with any other skill demanding manual dexterity, some people find more difficulty than others.

Another factor in the neglect of this branch of work by the medical profession has been the claims of manipulators that they were able to cure all manner of diseases by manipulation of the spine. This claim was so obviously unacceptable that it tended to blind the medical profession to what the manipulators were really doing. The reasons for this claim, and a possible explanation of it, are discussed in a later chapter. The effect of these extravagant claims was so to alienate the medical profession that its members were unprepared to accept anything that the manipulators said, nor were they even prepared to believe the patients who said they had benefited.

The general public is notorious for pursuing the unorthodox, even when experience later shows the stupidity of this action. In the case of manipulators, however, experience showed that the public could obtain genuine relief from the symptoms of spinal derangements by their treatment and this natural tendency to pursue the unorthodox was greatly reinforced. Because of this public demand, irregular practitioners have persisted and increased in numbers.

In the last 100 years two major schools of manipulative therapy have developed and their practitioners are widespread through many parts of the world. In spite of this, there are still large numbers of practising 'natural' manipulators, the successors to the old bone setters, and some of these may still be found without basic scientific training of any kind.

From time to time the voices of highly respected and competent doctors of medicine have been raised in favour of manipulative treatment, but until after the 1939–45 war, the number of such medical manipulators was small and they were generally despised by their colleagues.

One of the authors' (JFB) own early experiences highlight the scepticism and open prejudice displayed by members of the medical profession towards manipulative treatment. As a medical student at Oxford University he was encouraged to attend a special meeting of the Medical Society (Osler Society) which was addressed by a famous physician of the time, who, it now seems apparent in retrospect, attempted to prejudice his listeners against manipulators and their art. Later, when training at St Thomas' Hospital, London, where manipulative treatment was practised by Dr James Mennell in the physiotherapy department, and intending to enter the field of orthopaedic surgery, the author was strongly advised by the orthopaedic surgeons to avoid any contact with Dr Mennell's department. Even within his own hospital he (and later his successor Dr James Cyriax) was considered an outcast.

There has always been evidence available that patients have felt themselves to have been materially helped by manipulators and it seems therefore to be a pity that their work should be so readily condemned without even being investigated. Unfortunately, this type of criticism is only too common today.

Osteopathy

The two modern manipulative schools are undoubtedly successors to the old bone setters, in spite of their claims to have been started *ab initio* by their respective founders. The first of these was the osteopathic school which was founded by Andrew Taylor Still (1828–1917). Still was registered as a medical practitioner in Missouri, but some doubt has been cast on the quality of his training. According to Northup,[3] he entered Kansas City College of Physicians and Surgeons but, with the advent of the Civil War, dropped out of the course in order to enlist. His name does not appear in the catalogue of 1891 which lists the Kansas City College graduates up to that year. It appears that his training was completed by preceptorship, as, indeed, was that of most physicians in the United States at that time. Hildreth[4] reproduces a certificate of registration in Adair County in 1883 and another certificate dated 1893 which states that Still was on the roll of physicians and surgeons in Macon County as early as 1874.

According to Gevitz,[5] Still's education was partly at his father's side and from texts in anatomy, physiology and materia medica. At that time medical treatment tended to be brutal and Still became very dissatisfied. He had already started to question the validity of orthodox teaching before three of his family died of cerebrospinal meningitis in 1864 in spite of the best efforts of a fellow practitioner.

In about 1880 Still's ideas began to crystallise after his experience with a woman who came complaining of shoulder pain. He mobilised the spine and rib joints which relieved her pain but she came back later to tell him that it had also stopped the asthma from which she had suffered for a long time.

The American School of Osteopathy was founded by Still in 1892 and it is of interest that he was at that time registered as a physician. Gevitz suggested that in the early years at the school the training was not what would now be considered adequate.

According to Downing,[6] Still's interest started from a personal observation. He is said to have obtained relief from a severe headache by lying on his back with the upper neck supported by a rope slung between two trees.

Unfortunately, he antagonised the profession of his day by his attitude to them, by his shrewd business instinct and by his claims to cure all manner of disease.

The osteopathic profession in the United States has, during this century, made great strides forward. Doctors of Osteopathy are now equally licensed with Doctors of Medicine (MDs) throughout the USA and are trained in surgery of all kinds as well as in other specialties. Unfortunately, osteopathic colleges in other countries have not all achieved the same standard.

Chiropractic

The second manipulative school is that of chiropractic, which was started in 1895 in Davenport, Iowa, USA by D. D. Palmer who is described as a 'self-educated erstwhile grocer' in a book on chiropractic published in 1962.[7]

The start of chiropractic is said to date from a specific incident when Palmer manipulated the thoracic vertebrae of a Negro porter and by this means cured him of deafness from which he had suffered for some years. On the face of it, this is a fantastic and totally unacceptable claim. As a result of personal experience, however, there is no doubt in the mind of at least one of the authors that somatic dysfunction in joints in the upper thoracic spine can affect the function of the inner ear, presumably by way of its sympathetic innervation.

For the present argument, the fact that Palmer claims at that time to have manipulated a specific vertebra indicates at least a modicum of knowledge and experience of manipulative treatment. That incident is considered to be the starting point of chiropractic, but it is clear that Palmer must have been working on his ideas for some years before. It seems likely that he actually learned techniques from some other person, either a bone setter or an osteopath.

Like osteopathy, the art of chiropractic has spread far and wide, particularly in North America. This has happened in spite of the fact that even the more modern books on chiropractic contain passages which are nonsense to those grounded in the basic sciences of orthodox medicine.

It is well known that it is impossible to 'fool all the people all the time' and there is no doubt that a significant proportion of those who go to chiropractors for treatment receive benefit. The fact that their theories are unacceptable must not be allowed to blind the profession to this. It should, rather, be regarded as a challenge to the profession to develop adequate theories that will explain their successes and improve methods of achieving this success.

The need for and opposition to manipulative treatment

Industrial injuries in Canada are handled largely by a nationwide organisation of Workers Compensation Boards. One of the major problems which these boards have to handle is the large numbers of industrial injuries to the back. The results of orthodox treatment of these injuries have proved to be far from satisfactory, and most if not all of the provincial Workers Compensation Boards have authority to pay for chiropractic treatment in certain circumstances. The number of such treatments for which the boards can be held financially liable is strictly limited and the same is true of the prepaid medical insurance plans. This limitation reflects the general feeling of physicians that the chiropractic profession still lacks adequate overall ability to handle back problems well.

The attitude of the orthodox medical profession to anything 'strange' and 'new' has often been far from helpful and far from scientific. An editorial in the *British Medical Journal* in 1910[8] reads:

> In the sphere of medicine there is a vast area of 'undeveloped land' which Mr. Lloyd George has somehow failed to include in his Budget. It comprises many methods of treatment which are scarcely taught at all in the schools, which find no place in textbooks and which consequently the 'superior person' passes with gown uplifted to avoid a touch that is deemed pollution. The superior person is, as has more than once been pointed out, one of the greatest obstacles to progress.
>
> Rational medicine should take as its motto Molière's saying 'Je prends mon bien ou je le trouve'; whatever can be used as a weapon in this warfare against disease belongs to it of right . . . Now Dr. Bryce has witnessed the mysteries of osteopathy and tells us what he saw in a paper published in this week's issue . . . The results recorded by him are of themselves sufficient to justify us in calling attention to the method.
>
> Not to go so far back as Harvey, who was denounced by the leaders of the profession in his day as a circulator or quack, we need only recall how the open-air treatment of consumption was ridiculed when the idea was first put forward by Bebbington . . . famous physicians refused to listen to Pasteur because he was not a medical man; Lister was scoffed at; the laryngoscope was sneered at as a physiological toy; the early ovariotomists were threatened by colleagues with the coroner's court; electricity was looked upon with suspicion; massage, within one's own memory, was regarded as an unclean thing. But even now the vast field of physiotherapy is largely left to laymen for exploitation.

In an address to the Pacific Interurban Clinical Club, Dr Horace Gray[9] quoted Sir Robert Jones, nephew of Hugh Owen Thomas:

> . . . forcible manipulation is a branch of surgery that from time immemorial has been neglected by our profession, and as a direct consequence, much of it has fallen into the hands of the unqualified practitioner. Let there be no mistake, this has seriously undermined the public confidence, which has on occasion amounted to open hostility. If we honestly face the facts this attitude should cause us no surprise. No excuse will avail when a stiff joint,

which has been treated for many months by various surgeons and practitioners without effect, rapidly regains its mobility and function at the hands of an irregular practitioner. We should be self-critical and ask why we missed such an opportunity ourselves. The problem is not solved by pointing out mistakes made by the unqualified, the question at issue is their success. Reputations are not made in any walk of life simply by failures. Failures are common to us all and it is a far wiser and more dignified attitude on our part to improve our armamentarium than dwell upon the mistakes made by others.

As the result of representations by osteopaths wishing to obtain official licence in Great Britain, a Select Committee of the House of Lords prepared a report in 1935. Grave deficiencies were shown up in the practice of so-called osteopaths at that time and the Bill to recommend licensing was withdrawn by its sponsors. Recognition has still not been granted in spite of further attempts.

Timbrell Fisher[1] sums up a chapter in which he severely, but justly, criticises the osteopathic profession in England at that time.

> Space will not permit the dismal recital of some of the tragedies resulting from this method of treatment that have been observed. Yet it must be admitted that osteopaths sometimes effect cures in patients whose conditions have defied more traditional methods and it is of the utmost importance that we should face this fact squarely and endeavour to ascertain how these cures are brought about. These cases can be classified into three main categories, all of which really belong to the domain of manipulative treatment proper.
>
> In the first category are the patients whose symptoms are actually situated in the spinal column or back and in which the alleviation or cure is due to the breaking down of adhesions in ligament, muscle or aponeurosis.
>
> In the second category are the patients whose symptoms are not actually in the spine, but elsewhere, these symptoms being principally in the nature of a neurosis ... The simplicity of the theory, the conviction with which it is uttered and the actual treatment by spinal manipulation all act by powerful suggestion. Thus the osteopath may bring about a striking success although his explanation of its occurrence is erroneous.
>
> In the third category are the patients suffering from pains, often of a neuralgic nature, in various areas of the trunk or limbs. These are referred along with the distribution of the spinal nerves owing to some pressure at their vertebral exits, often due to rheumatism or the after-effects of injury. Familiar examples include many cases of occipital neuralgia due to pressure on the upper cervical nerve roots, some cases of brachial or intercostal neuritis causing pain in the extremities or chest, certain cases of obscure abdominal pain often wrongly diagnosed as due to some intra-abdominal lesion and many cases of sciatica due to pressure at the vertebral exits of the spinal nerve roots. Very many cases of such sciatic pain are caused by compression of the sciatic nerve roots by scar tissue due to early vertebral arthritis in the lumbar or lumbo-sacral regions. For many years the author has practised manipulation of the lumbar spine in this type of case, and, in his experience, the results are usually better than the orthodox immobilisation ...
>
> The osteopaths have also evolved the technique of manipulating the spine and of producing the maximum degree of movement between the individual vertebrae which is worthy of study ... As we have already seen the treatment of these conditions really belongs to the realm of manipulative treatment

proper, and the danger of building up a revolutionary system of medicine upon such a slender hypothesis, unsupported by scientific evidence, is so incalculable that it is our duty, as guardians of the public health to fight against this menace.

Progress

In England, because the osteopaths have not been licensed, the position they occupy in the eyes of the medical profession is similar to that which the chiropractors have in Canada. In North America osteopaths have for many years been licensed, permitted to prescribe drugs, perform surgery, run hospitals, sign death certificates and perform many of the other official duties which in England are only carried out by the orthodox medical profession. The fact that many osteopaths and chiropractors in England show clear evidence of continuing success, and the same is true of the chiropractors in North America, must be accepted as a considerable challenge to the allopathic medical profession. Without at least a reasonable proportion of success, even the gullibility of the public would not ensure prosperity.

Since the days of the House of Lords Select Committee in 1935, the osteopathic profession in England has gone a long way towards putting its house in order, both from the point of view of ethics and from that of sound scientific anatomy, physiology and pathology. Unfortunately, there remains a wide gap in their training so that they could not yet be considered for full medical qualification as has been achieved by the graduates of the American schools. A considerable mass of research has been done by the various schools of osteopathy, chiefly in the United States, but, unfortunately, much of this work still requires confirmation from other centres and it would be nice to see this done by the allopathic medical profession.

The chiropractic school has not yet achieved such a firm scientific foundation and, even in recent writings, theories are restated and claims made which are difficult or impossible to reconcile with what the medical profession reasonably considers to be established fact. In spite of this, many chiropractors have obtained, by training and experience, a sufficient knowledge of the vertebral column to be able to make a reasonable assessment of patients, to be aware of the major contraindications to manipulative therapy and to be able to perform manipulations in such a way that the patients are relieved. They still have a long way to go before they can reasonably be offered the degree of Doctor of Medicine, as was done for osteopaths in some of the American states.

It appears that outside the country it is not widely understood that, in the USA, doctors of osteopathy trained in American schools have exactly the same licence as MD physicians and that they share practices and work in the same hospitals.

The challenge

The existence at the present time in this field of three divergent schools of healing (in addition to others not specifically considered here) must be a source of concern to the medical profession. The orthodox profession is, without doubt, grounded on a very solid scientific foundation and must take pride of place. This fact does not exclude the possibility that the other schools may have something to offer and it is no less unreasonable to condemn them without further investigation than was the condemnation of Lister, Pasteur and so many others who introduced new ideas.

Unfortunately, our orthodox training tends to make us judge anything new by our existing practice and teaching, rather than by going back to basic anatomy, physiology and pathology, and it is always difficult to divest oneself of preconceived ideas.

The very success of the osteopaths and the chiropractors should be a stimulus to the orthodox medical profession to undertake an unbiased assessment of their ideas, methods and claims by those competent to do so. In this way alone can their merits be assessed and their good points incorporated into the teaching of medicine as a whole. So far most such investigations have been conducted in a thoroughly unscientific manner and have suffered from the start from a strong bias against the subject under investigation.

With the aid of modern diagnostic tools, including computer assisted tomography and magnetic resonance imaging, it ought to be possible to elucidate some of the basic problems which still remain unanswered in this field. Such research will, of course, require the expenditure of considerable sums of money and should be conducted in an area where independent observers can assess the effectiveness of both orthodox and unorthodox treatment given to patients in sufficient numbers to allow satisfactory analysis.

The medical profession claims that the healing art is its own exclusive province but, unfortunately, the general public does not agree. There will always be the 'odd man out' who will tend to seek treatment from an unorthodox practitioner for reasons that are often quite inadequate, but the present position is that many members of the public can obtain relief from unorthodox practitioners of manipulative therapy when they do not get the same relief from the orthodox profession.

What is the manipulator doing?

One of the patients relieved by the Dr Turner referred to in the preface was a woman still crippled by symptoms in spite of having had disc protrusions removed by one of the authors (JFB) at both L5–S1 and, later, L4–5. Dr Turner succeeded in relieving her by mobilising one of her sacroiliac joints and subsequent recurrences responded to similar treatments given by the author.

The suggestion that a sciatic radiation of pain could arise from the sacroiliac joint was difficult for the author to accept, believing as he then did that referred pain was due to direct interference with nerves or their roots. The results in this case and the author's subsequent experience have convinced him that a sacroiliac strain can indeed be a cause of a sciatic radiation of pain. No satisfactory proof of the mechanism of the pain reference has yet been demonstrated experimentally.

There are, of course, two joints in the spine which have no intervertebral disc, namely the occipitoatlantal and that between the 1st and 2nd cervical vertebrae. As the result of practical experience, the authors are also satisfied that joint derangements of both the occipitoatlantal and atlantoaxial joints can cause pain both locally and referred. These findings in the occipitoatlantal, atlantoaxial and sacroiliac joints strongly suggest that the disc itself is not the only important source of symptoms, and possibly not even the most important.

Many authors have arrived by similar means at similar conclusions and have developed theories of their own. Our own theories and the reasons for them will be discussed, but for the moment the manipulative techniques will be described on the basis that one is trying to put a stiffened joint through a range of movement, rather than anything more complicated.

Stiffness of the involved joints can be demonstrated both clinically and radiologically. The radiological demonstration requires a comparison of films taken in flexion and extension (or, but less easily, sidebending right and left) and, by this, it is possible to determine which joints are not moving at all and which have restricted motion. A knowledge of the normal range in the various joints and of the variations to be considered normal is, of course, essential.

The clinical demonstration depends on the appreciation of abnormalities of movement of spinal joints and tension differences in the soft tissues around them. These are more readily felt when the fingers have had considerable experience and this often makes the demonstration somewhat unconvincing to the newcomer. Initially the ligaments seemed of more interest, but now the muscles are the most important structures to evaluate. They are probably one of the main causes of both local and referred pain.

Some patients are very much easier to examine in this way than others. Severe obesity can make the examination very difficult, but, unfortunately, there is another group that is equally difficult. These are those people whose subcutaneous tissue is dense and fibrous so that it feels tough even when they are not unduly obese. The precise techniques are described later.

The techniques described are by no means new. Many of them were, in fact, described by Dr Thomas Marlin in 1934.[10] At that time he was in charge of what later became the physiotherapy department at University College Hospital, London, and he described in his introduction how he studied osteopathy at one of the colleges in the USA. He did this after finding that some of his patients had been relieved by manipulators even when he had failed to help them: 'The day is past when this form of treatment should be regarded as outside the scope of medical practitioners and this book is an attempt to present in readable form, some of those manipulations which I have learned.'

He also records that, after a demonstration of some of these techniques, one of his senior colleagues told him that some of them had been practised in England as long as 40 years before his demonstration.

Finally, a word of warning, issued by Mennell:[11] 'A simple locking of any of the joints may frequently be relieved by manipulation without anaesthetic though it is by no means everyone who is able to learn the requisite techniques . . . It is desirable that the people who fail to acquire the art of manipulation, however competent they may be otherwise, should realise their limitations and leave this branch of the work alone.'

In the years that have passed since this chapter was originally written a very large volume of research has been carried out. Unfortunately, some of the trials have been designed in a way that has proved of little value. Other trials have so specified the precise manipulation that is done (to all the participating patients) that the treatment has not been what was needed in many of the patients.

Even more sad is the fact that there is still an unwillingness on the part of many physicians to allow the possibility that treatment by manipulation (in the wide sense) can help some of the patients for whom they have no satisfactory answer themselves. The authors know of no controlled trial of surgery for back pain which gives any indication that it would be regarded as a good method of treatment in other fields. It is also a very much more expensive method than the outpatient visits required for manipulative treatment.

REFERENCES

1. Timbrell Fisher A. G. (1948). *Treatment by Manipulation*, 5th edn. London: Lewis.
2. Paget Sir James (1867). Cases that bone setters cure. *Brit. Med. J*; 1:1–4.
3. Northup G. W. (1936). *Osteopathic Medicine. An American Reformation.* Chicago: American Osteopathic Assn.
4. Hildreth A. G. (1938). *The Lengthening Shadow of Dr. Andrew Taylor Still.* Macon, Missouri: Hildreth.
5. Gevitz N. (1982). *The D.O.s, Osteopathic Medicine in America.* Baltimore: Johns Hopkins University Press.
6. Downing C. H. (1935). *Osteopathic Principles in Disease.* San Francisco: Orozco.
7. Homewood A. E. (1962). *The Neurodynamics of Vertebral Subluxation.* Publisher not cited.
8. Editorial (1910). *Brit. Med. J*; 2:638.
9. Gray H. (1938). Sacro-iliac joint pain. *Int. Clin*; 2:54–96.
10. Marlin T. (1934). *Manipulative Treatment.* London: Edward Arnold.
11. Mennell James (1945). *Treatment by Movement and Massage*, 5th edn. London: Churchill.

Chapter 2

Anatomy

Practitioners in their training acquire a basic working knowledge of the anatomy of the spinal column. The objects of this chapter are to refresh the reader's memory on points that he or she may have forgotten, to go into detail about specific points which are often neglected and to present some evidence suggesting that, in certain aspects, standard anatomical teaching is not fully in accord with recent research work.

It is the clinical experience of countless manipulators that patients obtain relief from certain symptoms after manipulation, not only of spinal joints themselves, but of the sacroiliac joints and, although this is perhaps not so commonly accepted, also of the costovertebral joints. In trying to understand the reasons for the success of manipulation, it is of fundamental importance that one should have an accurate picture of the structure and normal function of the joint concerned.

The classical paper of Mixter and Barr[1] stimulated the interest of the medical profession in the structure of the intervertebral joint. Since that time many papers have been published and a great deal of fundamental research has been carried out. Even so, it is important to remember the work that had gone before and an excellent review of this work is given by Armstrong[2] in his introduction.

THE SACROILIAC JOINT

In spite of much recent research work on the subject by anatomists, there remains in the minds of many physicians the idea that this joint is one in which no movement normally takes place. In many old editions of *Gray's Anatomy*, the joint is described as a diarthrodial joint but with the cartilage plates in close contact and partly united by patches of soft fibrocartilage and fine interosseous fibres.

Brooke[3] reported the results of the examination of 200 sacroiliac joints. He refers to the articular surface of the sacrum as being: 'flatly concaved from side to side, the concavity being most marked at the angle between the two limbs. Here the junction between the posterior and upper borders forms a prominent lip which fits into the corresponding depression behind the convex articular surface of the ilium. This constitutes an important interlocking mechanism around which rotation takes place.'

Brooke continues to describe the movement, which he says is slight but quite definite, and of both a gliding and rotatory nature. The gliding can be upwards, downwards, or backwards but the more important movement is rotatory and takes place around the interlocking mechanism of the middle segment which he described.

Brooke went on to say that in the infant and the pregnant woman the joint takes part in the movement of the lower spine, but he was unable, in his dissections, to find proof that it also occurs in non-pregnant adults.

With regard to the soft fibrocartilage and interosseous fibres described in the older editions of *Gray's Anatomy*, he says: 'Certainly in younger subjects of both sexes, the joint surfaces are quite smooth and separate and the presence of congenital fibrous strands bridging across the joint as described by Henri Vignes must be an extremely rare condition.' He concludes with the summary: 'The old description that the joint was an amphiarthrosis, was the description of a pathological change. The normal joint is of the diarthrodial type and in all probability takes part in movements backwards and forwards of the lumbar spine.

'The joint cavity itself is well defined with a continuous fringe of synovial membrane and, at times, the addition of an accessory limb. It is a diarthrodial joint, resembling in every characteristic any other joint of this type, becoming amphiarthrodial only under certain pathological conditions.'

In 1936 Pitkin and Pheasant published a series of papers on sacrarthrogenic telalgia.[4] This term they coined to describe 'a syndrome of pain which originates in the sacro-iliac and sacro-lumbar articulations and accessory ligaments. The referred pain affects gluteal and/or sacral regions and may affect any part or all parts of the lower extremities except the internal crural and plantar regions.'

They conclude:

1. that sacroiliac mobility can be demonstrated *in vivo* by measuring the movements of the ilia;
2. that in the standing position all motions of the trunk, with the exception of flexion and extension, are normally associated with unpaired antagonistic movements of the ilia about a transverse axis that passes through the centre of the symphysis pubis;
3. that rotation and lateral bending of the sacrum do not normally occur alone, but as correlated motions that are coincidental to antagonistic movements of the ilia.

They also state in their conclusions that sacrarthrogenic telalgia is not the result of irritation or compression of the trunks of peripheral nerves and, secondly, that abnormal sacroiliac mobility is a potent cause of abnormal ligament tension that produces this syndrome.

Horace Gray[5] discusses the detailed anatomy of the sacroiliac joint with a summary of the evidence for the existence of mobility. Describing both forward and backward torsion of the ilium on the sacrum, he expresses the opinion that: '. . . matching lumps and hollows need only move one millimeter and stick at the limit of normal motion to cause pain; and that this working hypothesis fits as well as any other hitherto offered to explain the clinical observation of pain in the back relieved abruptly by manipulation without anaesthetic.'

In the tenth edition of *Cunningham's Textbook of Anatomy*[6] the joint is described as a synovial joint but the surfaces are often irregular, causing a certain amount of interlocking between the facets. Movement is described as being greatly restricted by the irregularity of the articular facets and the thickness and disposition of the dorsal sacroiliac ligaments.

Weisl[7] investigated the movements of the sacroiliac joint by radiographic methods in the living subject. The pelvis was fixed in a special apparatus which also located the x-ray tube and cassette so as to produce comparable pictures. The position of the subject was then altered by various degrees of flexion and extension of the trunk and legs. Weisl reported the following findings.

> In a minority of subjects the sacral displacement was such that the sacral line remained parallel to its position at rest. Angular displacement occurred much more frequently and it was possible to locate an axis of rotation. It was situated approximately 10 cm below the promontory in the normal subjects, both recumbent and standing, and was placed a little higher in puerperal women. Contrary to the belief of previous authors, the site of this axis was variable in a majority of subjects, either the axis moved more than 5 cm following various changes of posture, or angular and parallel movement occurred in the same subject . . .
>
> The position of this axis of rotation differed from that described by earlier authors who based their opinions only on the examination of the sacro-iliac articular surfaces . . .

He also found that by these means there was no difference in the range of movement between males and females except in the puerperal state, and that difference in the range of movement could not be correlated with the height, weight or sacral curve index in the individual. The maximum constant movement was a ventral movement of the promontory of 5.6 ± 1.4 mm in the change of position from recumbency to standing. The movements on flexion and extension of the trunk were of smaller range and less consistent.

In recent editions of *Gray's Anatomy*[8] the sacroiliac joint is described as being a synovial joint and, in the adult, it is marked by a number of: '. . . irregular elevations and depressions. These irregularities, which are more pronounced in the male, fit into one another and provide a locking device restricting movement and contributing to the stability of the sacro-iliac joint . . . In the elderly, it is usual to find that the joint cavity is at least partly obliterated by the presence of fibrous or fibrocartilaginous adhesions and synostosis may occur. These changes are more common in the male.'

On applied anatomy, Gray describes the occurrence of sacroiliac strain with locking of the joints in the abnormal position, requiring forcible manipulation for its reduction. This is mentioned in connection with relaxation of the pelvic ligaments occurring in pregnancy.

There are striking differences in the conclusions drawn by Brooke, by Pitkin and Pheasant and by Weisl from their studies of the sacroiliac joint. The chief difference is in the location of the centre of movement of the joint and the findings are so far at variance as to suggest that, by the nature of their observations, one observer saw and measured one type of movement and another saw evidence of movement of a different type occurring at the same joint.

From the clinical point of view, the most important movement of the sacroiliac joint is one which may well have been excluded by the technique used by Weisl in his experiments. This is the antagonistic movement about a transverse axis through the symphysis pubis described by Pitkin and Pheasant. This movement cannot occur without producing torsion of the pelvis involving rotation of the ilia on the sacrum in opposite directions. Brooke[3] actually concluded that such torsional movements occur in the normal act of walking. Such rotations of ilium on sacrum could well occur around the interlocking mechanism of the middle segment described by Brooke. As a result of the innominate rotation the sacrum twists about its long axis so that the auricular surface faces more posteriorly on the side on which the innominate rotates, with the iliac crest becoming more posterior. The auricular surface on the same side is also tilted to face more caudally because of a small amount of rotation of the sacrum about an anteroposterior axis. This alteration of the position of the sacrum is, of course, transmitted to the superincumbent spine.

Fryette[9] points out that there are many anatomical variations in the sacrum. In particular he shows photographs of what he describes as the three main types.

Type A has the typical shape of the first segment. The dorsal transverse measurement is slightly greater than the ventral. This he finds is associated commonly with transverse (thoracic type) lumbosacral facet joints.

Type B has the dorsal transverse measurement of the first segment smaller than the ventral. The associated facets are sagittal (lumbar type).

Type C has one articular surface sloping out and the other in. In other words, one half of the sacrum is like type A and the other half like type B, with the corresponding facet joint alignments.

These observations suggest a further reason why pelvic joint dysfunction does not always follow a standard pattern.

The function of the three joints in the pelvic ring is probably the least well understood of any in the body. There is now no room for doubt that the sacroiliac joints are mobile, diarthrodial joints, although they have only a small range of movement. In the normal pelvis the symphysis pubis permits only twisting between the pubic bones. In the abnormal pelvis, however, other movements may occur including translation (upward on one side, downward on the other) and separation. This translation can sometimes be seen in the x-ray (Fig. 2.1). (See Kapandji[10] for an analysis of the effect of posture on the joints of the pelvis.) Rotation at the sacroiliac joint causing forward displacement of the pubic bone at the symphysis on the side upon which the individual is bearing his weight in standing was demonstrated by Schunke.[11]

The movement of the sacrum between the ilia is complex; it may rock in flexion and extension between the ilia or it may twist. The complexities and combinations which are found clinically defy any simple

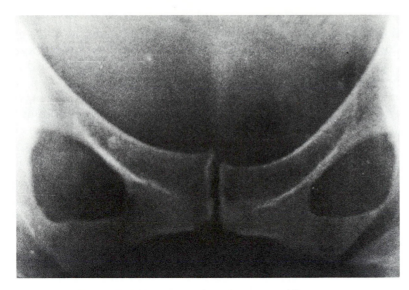

Fig. 2.1 Pubic symphysis showing subluxation.

mechanical explanation. While this difficulty at first bothers anyone who thinks about it, it is not really surprising. Evidence will be given later (see Chapters 12 and 13) which suggests that one of the problems with which we are primarily concerned is abnormal tension in muscle. A mechanical model which omits consideration of muscle function is not likely to give a full explanation.

The precise cause of the joint stiffness is still not known. Theories include persistent hypertonus in muscle, a mechanical loss of 'joint play', and entrapment of tissue between the joint surfaces. Although it is not the whole story, it is often helpful to think of the object of treatment as being to obtain relaxation of the muscle or muscles concerned and their associated soft tissues. The movements required to do this need not necessarily fit into a mechanical model which omits consideration of muscle function.

A twist of the pelvis produces an apparent inequality in the length of the legs and seriously affects the accuracy of the ordinary clinical methods of estimating any difference in leg length.

It will readily be appreciated that, if the pelvis has a fixed twist, the anterior superior spine will be higher on one side than on the other. Any measurement made from this point will then be in error by the amount of the difference in level.

Methods of estimating differences in leg length are described and discussed in Chapter 3 on examination.

The sacroiliac joints lie posterior to the coronal plane passing through the centre of the hip joints. If, therefore, the pelvis is twisted with the left innominate rotated backwards relative to the sacrum, the distance on the left side from the uppermost part of the sacral ala to the heel is reduced.

This alteration in effective leg length by movement of the sacrum is illustrated in Fig. 2.2. With the subject erect, an alteration in the angular position of the sacroiliac joint will cause an alteration in the angle made by a fixed line on the innominate bone with the horizontal (the only alternative would be tilting of the spine forwards or backwards out of the erect posture). This alteration in the tilt of the innominate bone will, of course, produce a change in the angle *theta*. This is the angle between a vertical dropped from the centre of movement of the hip joint and a line joining that centre of movement to a fixed part of the sacroiliac joint. The position of the centre of movement as described by Brooke is used for convenience. Simple geometry shows that when the angle *theta* is reduced, the distance between the floor and the fixed point on the sacroiliac joint is also reduced, producing an apparent shortening of the limb.

Differences in actual leg length of the lower limb are common. In the majority the differences are minor, being less than 7 mm (0.25 inch). Differences in leg length of more than 7 mm are not uncommon and can, of course, result from malunion of fractures or from other pathological changes in the lower limbs. Leg inequality is sometimes familial and, in these cases, the difference may well be 13 mm (0.5 inch) or more.

In patients with leg inequality there is a natural tendency for the pelvis to adopt the twisted position which most nearly levels the anterosuperior surface of the sacrum. This means that on the side of the longer leg, the sacroiliac joint will habitually adopt a posture with the innominate rotated posteriorly with respect to the sacrum. Unfortunately the stresses and strains of life tend to cause the sacroiliac joint to stiffen in that position, the more so if the subject is engaged in a heavy occupation. Simple

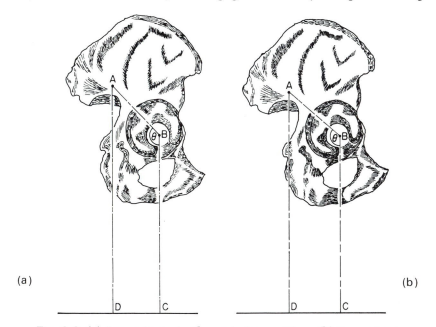

(a)

(b)

Fig. 2.2 (a) Innominate in the anterior position. **(b)** Innominate in the posterior position. The line B–C remains the same length but A–D has become shorter.

stiffness of the sacroiliac is not necessarily a cause of symptoms but it can easily become so and an example is a patient who suffered from acute low back pain. She had had a below knee amputation of her right leg 10 years before and was wearing a prosthesis which appeared to be too long. Treatment of the sacroiliac joint by manipulation gave her relief but the pain tended to return until she had the length of the prosthesis corrected. X-ray measurement of the leg length difference when wearing the limb showed that it was 2.5 cm (1 inch) too long.

In a person with an actual difference in the length of the lower limbs, the adoption by the pelvis of the twisted position will diminish the tilting of the sacrum. Unfortunately, the backward movement of the innominate on one side and the forward movement on the other causes a rotation of the sacrum about its long axis. This rotation is, of course, transmitted to the lumbar spine. It seems probable that there is a righting mechanism which tends to correct the rotation higher in the spine in order to preserve the forward pointing attitude of the head. This twist, and the corrective forces which it causes, tend to predispose the patient to trouble in the spine above. The reason for this is, apparently, that a joint which is held in an 'off-centre' position for any length of time will tend to become stiff and associated with hypertonus in muscle.

For this reason, observation of leg length difference is most important in patients complaining of back symptoms. If a difference is found in excess of 7 mm (0.25 inch), a correction by means of an alteration to the shoe is frequently necessary. If the leg length difference continues unobserved and uncorrected, the constant (if minor) strain which it produces may make it difficult or impossible to cure the lumbar symptoms.

If a fixed pelvic twist occurs as a result of injury in a patient with equal legs, the effect on the lumbar spine is essentially similar. The rotatory displacement of the sacrum about its long axis is the same, but there is now a tilting of that long axis towards the side on which the innominate is in the posterior position. In a case of leg length difference where the difference is too great to be fully corrected by the pelvic twist, the tilt of the sacral long axis is, of course, in the opposite direction. In either case, recognition and treatment of the pelvic dysfunction may be of vital importance in the care of the patient.

In this connection it may be worth restating the author's (JFB) feeling of blank disbelief at the first mention of the sacroiliac joint as a cause of back and leg pain. This disbelief arose from the idea, still paramount in the minds of many physicians, that referred leg pain was caused by actual pressure on nerves or nerve roots. Although entrapment neuropathy may give rise to such pain, that referred from the sacroiliac joint is not, as far as has been determined, due to physical entrapment.

The sacroiliac joint has one other characteristic in which it is different from the intervertebral joints and which is important from a clinical point of view. This is the absence of easily palpable muscle crossing and controlling the joint, so that there is no muscle in which hypertonus is diagnostic. Some increase in muscle tension over the upper two sacral segments is commonly found however.

Diagnosis, therefore, depends primarily on asymmetry and loss of

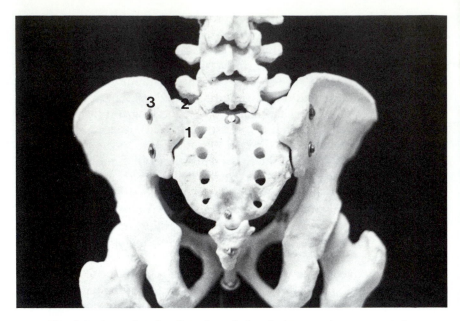

Fig. 2.3 Articulated pelvis from behind. (For explanation of the figures, see the text.)

movement. The finding of hypertonus in the lowest segments of the erector spinae will help when present, so also will tenderness over the posterior sacroiliac ligament. The clinical finding that symptoms are still present after adequate treatment of the lumbar joints may alert the examiner to a previously unobserved sacroiliac joint dysfunction. Methods of detection of loss of movement between the sacrum and the ilia and for determining the relative position of the bones will be described in the chapters on examination.

With respect to the finding of tenderness, it is important to distinguish between tenderness of the posterior sacroiliac ligament, found medial to the lower part of the posterior superior spine (Fig. 2.3, 1), and the tender area very commonly found on the back of the ilium lateral to the posterior superior spine (Fig. 2.3, 3). The latter is usually caused by hypertonus in the origin of the gluteal muscles. It may result from dysfunction of joints anywhere in the lumbar spine. It is important to remember that tenderness medial to the superior part of the posterior spine is more likely to be associated with lumbosacral problems (Fig. 2.3, 2).

Before leaving the sacroiliac joint, mention must be made of Baer's sacroiliac point, described many years ago. It is a tender point occurring in the right iliac fossa just medial to McBurney's appendix point. It is described as being tender when infection involves the right sacroiliac joint but may also be found in acute strains of that joint.

SPINAL BALANCE

The concept that the spinal column should be regarded as a single functional unit is at variance with clinical teaching, in spite of the fact that there appears to have been no attempt from within the profession to develop or to learn a method of examining the individual spinal joint as a separate entity. It has already been shown that a sacroiliac fixation resulting in twisting of the pelvis can, and does, cause a disturbance of function in the lumbar region. Experience shows that if a joint becomes stiffened at one end of its travel in the lumbar region, a disturbance of function tends to occur at other levels above and below. This also applies to stiffness occurring primarily either in the thoracic or in the cervical spine. If, for instance, the second lumbar vertebra is forced into the extreme of sidebending and rotation to the right, so that the joint between the 2nd and 3rd lumbar vertebrae becomes stiffened in this position, the natural tendency of the spine to adopt a corrective posture will result in the opposite deformity at one or more joints either above or below the lesion.

Again drawing on clinical experience, one finds that unless the primary lesion is relieved, the joints which are secondarily affected will in time tend to stiffen and in many cases will start producing symptoms. These secondary symptom-producing joints are most commonly found in the lower thoracic region, at the cervicothoracic junction, in the upper cervical spine, or at the joint above or below the original lesion. When the secondary joints do become stiff, they tend themselves to be the cause of a third generation of levels of joint dysfunction, usually at a greater distance from the original lesion. Patients are often seen in whom the primary levels of dysfunction are no longer producing symptoms. The problem here is that the secondary symptom-producing joints will probably continue to give trouble, however well they are treated, if the primary joint problem is not also corrected.

These considerations suggest that a difference in leg length can be a predisposing cause to persistent trouble from stiffened joints, even in the cervical region.

In his training the author (JFB) was taught to regard as seriously neurotic any patient who complained of pain which started in the low back and ran up the back and down the arm. The basis of this teaching was that no single cause could produce this symptom complex. Considerations of the functional interdependence of the parts of the spine suggest that the symptom complex can have a real organic basis in multiple joint dysfunction. In such a patient muscle spasm, produced at one level by a further strain, could well cause sufficient upset of the joints at other levels for symptoms to arise from these also.

THE PHYSIOLOGICAL MOVEMENTS OF THE SPINAL COLUMN

Kapandji[12] describes the automatic rotation of the vertebral column during lateral flexion but does not mention the differences which depend on the degree of flexion or extension of that segment of the spine.

The original observation appears to have been made by Lovett[13] when working on the problem of scoliosis. He found that a column of vertebral bodies separated from its posterior elements behaved as in Kapandji's description. If the column is sidebent, the bodies rotate to the convexity of the sidebend. When he examined the column of posterior elements, however, the rotation was always to the concavity of the sidebend.

Lovett described that, with the intact spine in the living model or the cadaver, the rotation varied. With the spine in extension the rotation was towards the concavity of the sidebend. With the spine flexed the rotation was to the convexity.

Lovett also showed that in extension the facets were held in close apposition but this was not the case in flexion. He concluded that in extension the facets exert a controlling influence because of their close apposition to each other.

Fryette[9] showed that while Lovett's observations were correct, he had omitted to test the movements in the hyperflexed position. Near the limit of flexion the pattern changes once again. The facets assume control and the rotation once again is in the direction of the concavity of the sidebend. These findings were formulated by Fryette into the two laws of spinal motion and this concept has found wide acceptance in the osteopathic profession. For completeness a third law is added.

Law I With the spine in easy flexion (neutral), the facets are idling and the rotation is always to the convexity of the sidebend.

Law II In extension and in nearly full flexion, the facets are in control and the rotation must be to the concavity of the sidebend.

Law III If movement is introduced into a spinal segment in any plane, the range of movement in the other two planes will be reduced.

The clinical significance of this is that there is a cross-over point where the rotation reverses. If, for instance, one bends to reach the floor and then twists sideways, one is in danger of 'jamming' the mechanism if one tries to come up quickly without first undoing the twist. This, indeed, is one of the ways of producing acute back pain.

When the joint becomes jammed with the rotation into the concavity of the curve, i.e. in accordance with the second law of spinal motion, it is known as a Type II lesion. Such lesions are commonly traumatic, usually quite acute, and should be treated first. The causative trauma will have occurred either in extension or in hyperflexion of the spine.

When the joint becomes held in a position where rotation is to the convexity of the curve (in accordance with Law I), it is known as a Type I lesion. These are often compensatory and may resolve when the primary joint is treated. Such lesions occur in groups while Type II lesions are nearly always solitary.

In using the words 'jammed' or 'held' the authors do not wish to beg the question as to which comes first, the stiffness of the joint or the tightness of the muscle.

THE INTERVERTEBRAL JOINTS

The spinal joint stiffness referred to above is demonstrable both by palpation and by special radiographic techniques. The anatomical and pathological basis for this stiffening is still not agreed. Careful examination of x-rays indicates that in the ordinary sense of the word, there is no displacement. Recent workers have suggested that the explanation may be connected with the intra-articular structures which exist in the facet joints throughout the spine. The existence of these structures has been known for many years but there has been some argument as to their nature and importance.

Schmincke and Santo[14] in 1932 gave a clear description of structures in the cervical region which they considered to be true intra-articular 'discs'.

Santo[15] later described two different types of structure in the thoracic and lumbar regions, one thin and vascular, the other fibrous with some cartilage cells. He regarded the former as a synovial fold and the latter as an articular 'disc'.

Tondury[16] described similar structures and regarded them as derived from the synovial membrane, but he also found a connection between some of the structures and the extra-articular pad of fat.

Zaccheo and Reale[17] investigated 20 vertebral columns from infancy to old age and described three different types of intra-articular structures, including not only those described by Schmincke, Santo and Tondury but also what they consider to be a true meniscus. The other structures they described as synovial folds and fatty bodies respectively.

They regard the meniscus as having the typical functions of shock absorption and padding to produce conformity of shape on movement. The other structures are thought to be concerned with production of synovial fluid and with the filling up of spaces left above and below the joint on flexion movement.

It seems conceivable that injury to these structures, small as they are, could result in an upset of joint function and be responsible for symptoms.

Dorr[18] also studied the anatomy of the intervertebral joint in detail and described similar structures as well as interlaminar bursae found in the cervical region. He discusses the function of the various structures and concludes: 'We were unable to discover from our studies whether "trapped discs" are the cause of backache' (author's translation), but goes on to compare them with the menisci in the knee joint and deduces that if a meniscus is first trapped by positioning and then moved, it could cause pain by traction on the capsule.

Lewin *et al.*[19] review the literature and describe further investigations into the anatomy of the intervertebral joint. They point out that the meniscus-like structures are in fact true menisci because they are found at all ages, including in the newborn. They point to the lack of synovial cells over the majority of the surface of the menisci as an indication that these structures actually bear weight.

Lewin and his co-workers also investigated the movements and point out that the intervertebral joint must be regarded as a triad consisting of the disc and the two apophyseal joints. On flexion and extension the facets slide in the sagittal plane while the nucleus displaces dorsally or ventrally, on sidebending the facets slide in opposite directions and the nucleus displaces away from the direction of flexion: 'If any rotation occurs in the lumbar spine, it happens in spite of the fact that the lumbar joints are designed to prevent rotation ... an attempt to impose a rotatory movement on the lumbar spine subjects the lumbar joints to their greatest loading and at the same time exerts a shearing moment on the intervertebral disc.'

In view of this finding, it is interesting to note that for many years the usual movement performed for lumbar joint dysfunction has involved rotation. This is described later, as are other methods (see Chapters 8 and 9).

It is an observed fact that treatments directed towards obtaining relaxation of the abnormally tight muscle can in some circumstances be highly successful. This success suggests that one of the main factors in producing and maintaining the loss of motion in the joint is the abnormal tension in the muscle.

THE DISC

The annulus is composed of rings of fibrocartilage, 18 to 20 in number in an adult, set at an angle to each other. Posteriorly, the lamellae run vertically and are parallel bands, but at their lateral extremities they are interlaced with the oblique fibres. In infants the lamellae are less distinct and fewer in number, but become more clearly differentiated and increase in numbers until about the end of the growth period. Increase in thickness of the annulus is partly at the expense of the nucleus and partly by appositional growth from the long ligaments.[20] The ends of the fibres forming the lamellae are firmly attached to the bone and in front are reinforced by the strong anterior common ligament. Both above and below the disc, these fibres tend to curl inwards around the nucleus before being attached to the bone. The unaltered nucleus is not a pulp, but a translucent gel containing a three-dimensional network of fine collagen fibrils.[21]

Hirsch[22] found that the nucleus 'is not a watery gel but is composed of highly organised material'. He also described numerous collagen fibres in the nuclei of children and young persons surrounded by chondromucoid elements. Hirsch and Schajowicz[20] found radiating ruptures in many autopsy discs. When complete they contained highly vascular connective tissue which had grown out from the long ligament. Concentric cracks or cavities were even more common but were thought to be physiological.

In normal discograms Lindblom[23] showed that the disc contained cavities which could be filled with contrast medium. These cavities were principally above and below the nucleus, between it and the vertebral end-plates. In the abnormal the cavity was more extensive, extending backwards close to the vertebra. This was apparently caused by tearing of the fibres attaching the annulus to bone and resulted from loss of elasticity of the posterior annulus secondary to the radiating cracks which appear in degenerating discs.

The avascularity of the disc has been commented on by many workers and appears to be complete except for the most superficial part of the annulus.[2] No nerve fibres have been demonstrated in the disc other than by Roofe,[24] who found them in the posterior part of the annulus. These appear to arise from the sinuvertebral nerve of Luschka.

THE OCCIPITOATLANTAL AND ATLANTOAXIAL JOINTS

The structure and function of the intervertebral joints from the lumbosacral up to that between the 2nd and 3rd cervical are essentially similar throughout, although there are marked individual variations in the range of motion. In the thoracic region there is the added complication of the neighbouring costovertebral articulations with their associated muscles and ligaments. Between the skull and the 1st cervical and between the 1st and 2nd cervical vertebrae there is a profound change in structure which is necessitated by the change in function at this level. The occipitoatlantal joint is designed to give a maximum of flexion and extension movement in the sagittal plane with some sidebending. Werne[25] investigated the movement of the occipitoatlantal and atlantoaxial joints and concluded that rotatory movement did not occur at the occipitoatlantal nor did tilting to the side occur at the atlantoaxial joint (but see Kapandji[10]). He said that the two joints should be regarded as a functional unit permitting flexion and extension at the upper and, to a less extent, at the lower joint and permitting sidebending at the upper joint and rotation at the lower joint. He did, however, conclude that 'tilting and turning are always combined' even if they occur at separate anatomical sites. Fielding[26] points out that vertical approximation is also possible at the occipitoatlantal joint.

In neither joint is there an intervertebral disc, nor is there any other structure that can cause actual pressure on nerve or nerve root in a confined space, as can happen in a typical intervertebral joint with a posterolateral disc protrusion.

Similarly, in the sacroiliac joint there can be no question of nerve pressure from a disc protrusion. The symptoms and signs which can only be produced by actual nerve compression therefore do not occur in lesions of these three joints. Stiffness, local pain and referred pain and tenderness can and do occur, and are comparable in every respect to the similar symptoms arising in typical intervertebral joints.

THE INNERVATION OF THE INTERVERTEBRAL JOINTS

The innervation of the structures of and around the intervertebral joints was investigated by Pedersen *et al.*[27] and more recently by Wyke.[28] Their findings are basically similar. Wyke described:

1. branches of the posterior primary rami supplying the apophyseal joints, the periosteum and the related fasciae of the surfaces of the vertebral bodies and their arches, the interspinous ligaments and the blood vessels;

2. pain afferents in the sinuvertebral nerves having endings in the posterior longitudinal and flaval ligaments, the dura mater and the surrounding fatty tissue, the epidural veins and the periosteum of the spinal canal;

3. a plexus of nerve fibres which surrounds the paravertebral venous system. Receptors supplied by these nerves are found throughout the same area as those supplied by the sinuvertebral nerve. All the pain afferent fibres are small, either thinly or not at all myelinated.

THE MUSCLES OF THE SHOULDER GIRDLE AND UPPER TRUNK

The muscles of the upper back are arranged in three groups.[29] The superficial group comprises the muscles connecting the shoulder girdle to the trunk and consists of the trapezius, latissimus dorsi, levator scapulae, and the rhomboids. These have all migrated caudalwards and their innervation is derived from cervical segments. Tender areas in these muscles can, therefore, be expected to be associated with disturbances of cervical nerve function. The intermediate group consists of the serratus posterior superior (and inferior). These are muscles of respiration which have migrated backwards. They are innervated by the ventral rami of the thoracic nerves and deep to these are the muscles of the spinal column itself which are innervated by the dorsal rami. Any disturbance of the intermediate or deep muscles can therefore be expected to be associated with an alteration in function of the thoracic, rather than cervical, nerves.

The clinical importance of this is that muscle tenderness between the midline and the vertebral border of the scapula up to the back of the first rib can, if superficial, be due to a cervical joint disturbance or, if deep, to trouble in the thoracic spine. The distinction of the depth at which the muscle is tender may be difficult to make and therefore the examination must include both cervical and thoracic regions.

RANGE OF MOBILITY OF INDIVIDUAL SPINAL JOINTS

Cervical

Measurement of the range of flexion–extension movement in the individual cervical joints has been undertaken by a number of authors. Penning[30] gives the figures quoted by several authors, including himself, describes his technique and discusses the results. The technique he used was to take lateral radiographs in the fully flexed and fully extended positions of the neck and a third view with the head fully flexed on the neck, but the neck itself only partly flexed. This was necessary because he found that full flexion of the neck tended to cause a deflexion at the occipitoatlantal joint in order to get the chin out of the way. The

Table 2.1 Range of Sagittal Motion in the Cervical Spine (Penning)

Joint	Range in degrees	Average
Co–1	6 to 30	—
C1–2	3 to 35	—
C2–3	5 to 16	$12\frac{1}{2}$
C3–4	13 to 26	18
C4–5	15 to 29	20
C5–6	16 to 29	$21\frac{1}{2}$
C6–7	6 to 25	$15\frac{1}{2}$
C7–T1	4 to 12	8

measurement of the angle of movement was done by superimposing each vertebra in turn and marking the film in a similar way to that described by Troup[31] for the lumbar spine.

Penning's average results are very similar to those of other recent workers, but the range of individual variation is great in all the series published. The results obtained by Penning himself are set out in Table 2.1.

Thoracic

Motion is restricted in the thoracic region in all directions when compared to either of the other regions. There appear to have been no experimental studies of the range of movement of the individual joints. There is a relatively abrupt change in mobility between the C6–7 and the T1–2 joints, but a major part of this change occurs between the C6–7 and the C7–T1 joints, Penning's average movement for the latter being only half the average of the former.

The transition at the thoracolumbar junction takes place at a joint which differs structurally from both the thoracic joint above and the lumbar joint below. The structural difference lies in the shape of the articular processes which, at this level, have been likened by Davis[32] to a carpenter's mortice. This joint is most commonly found between the 11th and 12th thoracic but can be either at that between T10 and T11 or, rather more commonly, at that between T12 and L1. Owing to the shape of the articular processes at this level, movements other than flexion–extension are much restricted and flexion–extension is also less free than at any of the joints below.

Lumbar

A very full discussion of the literature and fresh experimental work are reported by Troup.[31] He examined statistically a variety of different methods of measuring the movement between individual lumbar vertebrae as shown by x-rays in the flexed and in the extended position.

By statistical analysis, Troup was able to show that a method of marking angles by successive superimposition of the outlines of the individual lumbar vertebrae was very significantly superior to any of the methods which involve the drawing of lines on the films to mark the inclination of the individual vertebrae. The method of superimposition of x-rays was originally described by Begg and Falconer[33] and was that used by Penning for the cervical spine.

Most other workers who have recorded the range of movement of the lumbar spine by radiological methods have relied on the measurement of angles between lines drawn on the x-rays designed to show the inclination of the individual vertebra. The inaccuracy appears to be due in part to the difficulty in determining the exact position of the points between which the line should be drawn and in part to the fact that a double error is involved as for each measurement two lines have to be drawn.

In Troup's modification of Begg and Falconer's superimposition method, the outlines of the sacrum on the two x-rays are first superimposed. The x-rays are, of course, taken in the lateral projection, one with the spine flexed and the other with it extended. Care must be taken to see that the relationships of the tube head, pelvis and cassette are standardised.

With the two sacra superimposed, a line is drawn on the underneath film marking one of the edges of the upper film. The upper film is then realigned so that the outlines of the 5th lumbar vertebrae are superimposed. A second line is then drawn marking the same edge of the upper film on the film underneath, and the process is repeated for each of the lumbar vertebrae. Finally, the angles between the successive lines are measured with a protractor.

Troup[31] points out that the exposure to radiation involved in taking films of the lumbar spine is sufficient to be a hazard, the more so because of the proximity of the sex glands. He therefore regarded the method as unjustified in the normal and the figures which he gives are based on radiographic examination of patients with lumbar symptoms for whom this was needed on clinical grounds. It is likely, therefore, that his figures are somewhat lower than would be obtained by a similar examination of strictly normal spines.

The means and standard deviations of the estimated movements of the individual joints in Troup's series are set out in Table 2.2.

Table 2.2 Range of Sagittal Motion in the Lumbar Spine (Troup)

Joint	Full flexion to full extension		Full flexion to erect position	
	Mean	*SD*	*Mean*	*SD*
L1–2	7.5	2.3	8.6	1.7
L2–3	10.5	3.4	10.3	3.6
L3–4	11.1	2.8	11.2	2.5
L4–5	12.9	4.0	12.0	3.9
L5–S1	11.0	3.9	9.0	6.4

Table 2.3 Range of Sagittal Motion in the Lumbar Spine (Froning and Frohman)

Number of cases	Ages	L5	L4	L3	L2	L1
5	20–29	18	17	14	14	13
11	30–39	17	16	14	10	9
8	40–49	16	16	13	10	8
5	50–59	16	15	12	11	7
1	60–70	16	14	10	10	6
	Average	17	16	13	11	9

A somewhat surprising result shown in Troup's figures is that in the upper two lumbar joints there is a tendency for a flexor movement to occur between the erect and the fully extended posture of the body. In some subjects there was a flexor movement in the upper two lumbar joints when the spine was extended beyond the erect position. This can be compared to the deflexion of the occipitoatlantal joint mentioned above.

Also in 1968, Froning and Frohman[34] investigated the range of movement at the individual lumbar joints in patients and in people with supposedly normal spines. The figures for the normal are reproduced in Table 2.3 and it will be seen that the figures for the L4–5 and L5–S1 joints are significantly greater than those given by Troup.

Troup's observations were on those with lumbar symptoms and it is well known that such symptoms more commonly arise from the lower two lumbar joints than from the upper three. It is, therefore, to be expected that Troup's figures for patients with symptoms would be lower, particularly with respect to the L4–5 and L5–S1 joints, than those obtained from supposedly normal people. The requirements for normality as laid down by Froning and Frohman were a balanced standing posture, negative neurological findings, absence of sciatic nerve tenderness or pain on stretching the nerve and no x-ray changes either in the osseous structures or in the disc spaces. They point out that the numbers in the various age groups are small owing to the difficulty in obtaining a sufficient number who fulfilled these strict conditions. A striking conclusion to be drawn from these figures is that among those who fulfil these criteria for normality, the loss of motion with increasing age is remarkably slight.

In their study of abnormal spines, Froning and Frohman found that a significantly increased range of motion was common in joints adjacent to those showing restriction. Jirout[35] recorded similar results and this finding may explain the clinical observation of restricted motion in individual joints in a part of the spine with normal overall mobility.

Froning and Frohman also found that after partial disc removal a statistically significant proportion of cases with good results showed restriction of motion but those with bad results retained greater mobility. The reasons for this were not discovered.

For a full discussion of the physiology of the joints of the spine see

Kapandji,[10] but note that he appeared to be unaware either of Penning's observations on movements of the occipitoatlantal joints or of Froning and Frohman's observations on lumbar movements in the normal ageing spine.

THE AUTONOMIC NERVOUS SYSTEM

The precise role of both sympathetic and parasympathetic nerves in the appreciation of pain remains to be worked out. Experience with many clinical cases indicates that pain reference often occurs from certain spinal segments to parts of the body with which that segment appears to have no nerve connection other than in the autonomic system. Bingham[36] thought that there was evidence that pain actually travelled in sympathetic afferent fibres. The problem is discussed by Barnes,[37] who concludes that it is unlikely on the following grounds.

1. No sensory change of any kind has ever been demonstrated in a sympathectomised limb.

2. In cord lesions where the cord is damaged below the lowest sympathetic outflow, the sympathetic innervation of the lower limbs is intact but there is a total insensibility of the area supplied by somatic nerves arising in segments below the damage.

3. A low spinal anaesthetic will relieve the pain of causalgia before there is any effect on the sympathetic fibres.

On clinical grounds alone there is ample evidence to show that some disturbance of sympathetic function can be associated with the production of referred pain in certain sites. Therefore, the level of origin of sympathetic fibres to various parts of the upper and lower limbs is of interest to the surgeon who is called upon to find the source of certain types of referred pain. The level of the sympathetic outflow supplying the head, neck and trunk is generally better known, but that to the head is included because it seems likely that abnormal sympathetic activity is one of the major factors in the production of some headaches and, if these are the result of a spinal joint abnormality, it is important to know at which level to look (Table 2.4).

Mitchell[38] states that afferent pain fibres from the cervix uteri, base of bladder, prostate and rectum are carried in the pelvic splanchnic nerves and their cells are located in the dorsal root ganglia of the 2nd, 3rd and 4th sacral nerves.

Neuwirth[39] reviews relatively recent work on the anatomy of the sympathetic nervous system, most of which was done in France by Laruelle,[40] Delmas *et al.*,[41] and Tinel.[42] Laruelle describes his demonstration of sympathetic cell bodies in the mediolateral grey matter at the base of the anterior horns at the levels of the spinal cord segments of C4, 5, 6, 7 and 8. The preganglionic fibres from these are said to proceed with the somatic motor fibres in the ventral roots from C5 to T1 inclusive, and are said to synapse in the small ganglia found on the sympathetic plexus around the vertebral artery. Others traverse these

Table 2.4 Sympathetic Innervation of More Important Structures (based on Mitchell)

Structure	Location of pre-ganglionic cells	Chief efferent pathways
Eyes	T1–2	Internal carotid plexus to ciliary nerves or along vessels
Vessels of head	T1–2 (and 3)	Vascular plexuses
Upper limbs	T2(3) to T6(7)	Rami communicates to roots of brachial plexus
Heart	T1–4(5)	Cardiac sympathetic nerves to cardiac plexus
Stomach	T6–9(10)	Via coeliac plexus
Kidneys	T12(11) to L1(2)	Via coeliac plexus
Bladder and uterus	T12(11) to L1(2)	Lumbar splanchnic nerves
Lower limbs	T11(10) to L2	Rami communicates to lumbar and sacral nerves

ganglia, join the plexus and by this means reach the cervicothoracic group. According to Tinel, the fibres of C5 join the carotid plexus and are distributed to the subclavian plexus and thereby reach the arm and the nerves of the brachial plexus. Those from C7 go to the cardio-aortic plexus, to the thoracic branches of the axillary and subclavian arteries and the phrenic nerves.

By these findings Neuwirth sought to explain:

1. the relief of headaches and facial pain which can follow treatment of the neck;

2. similar results with what he terms dysaesthesias and vascular pain in the upper extremity; and

3. pain in the upper part of the back and anterior chest wall simulating angina.

Unfortunately, this work, which was done in France, has not yet been confirmed by other workers. The volume of the sympathetic outflow at these levels appears to be small and it seems likely that the true explanation involves some other nervous mechanism.

SENSORY DISTRIBUTION OF THE SPINAL NERVE ROOTS

It has been known for many years that the distribution of sensory fibres to the skin from the various spinal nerve roots does not correspond to the distribution of any of the cutaneous nerves, except over the trunk where the correspondence is fair. Head[43] studied the distribution of the cutaneous hyperalgesia and the vesicles in cases of herpes zoster. As a result of this study he was able to draw a map showing the distribution of the various spinal nerves with respect to the skin of the body. At about the same time Sherrington[44] mapped the distribution of nerve fibres by a different technique.

Sherrington worked with the rhesus monkey which, at least in the head, neck, upper limbs and trunk, has a very similar nerve distribution to that of man. In his experiments the posterior roots of a number of nerves were cut on either side of the one under investigation. The sensation remaining was then mapped by means of a painful stimulus applied to the area, note being made of a minimal motor response. The chief difference between the results obtained by Sherrington and those obtained by Head lay in the fact that Sherrington's areas were considerably larger and indicated major overlap, whereas Head's were discrete, with almost no overlap.

The configuration of the lumbar spine is different in the rhesus monkey and the human, and there appears to be some difference in the distribution of the lumbar and sacral nerves to the lower limbs so that the correspondence of the areas in the lower limb is less good. Both Head and Sherrington found that the areas which were mapped in the more distal parts of the limb were separated from the spine by skin which apparently

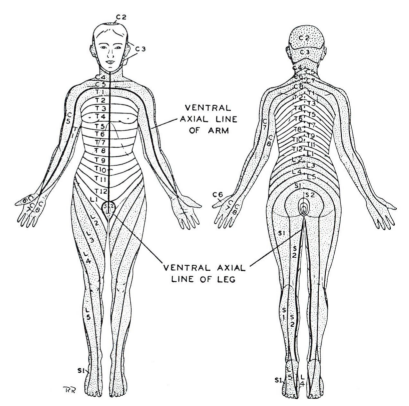

Fig. 2.4 Dermatome chart of the human body drawn by Keegan and Garrett.

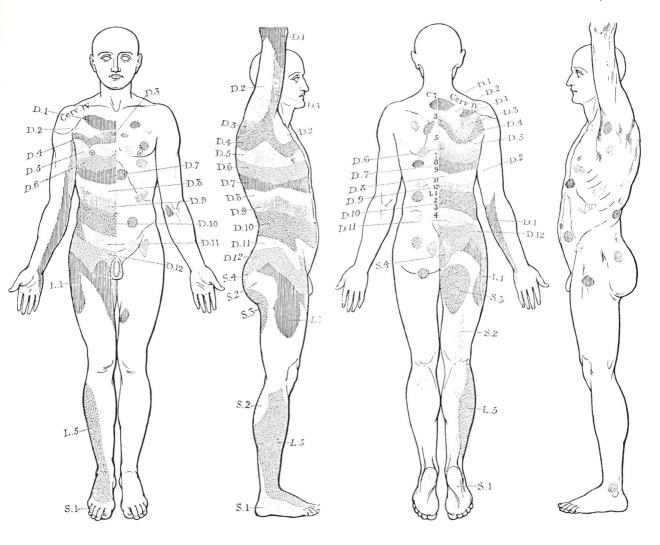

Fig. 2.5 Dermatome chart drawn by Head, showing both the total
area and the maxima.

had no sensory innervation from the spinal segment under investigation.
This led to the belief that the growing limb bud drew away from the
trunk all the sensory supply of the nerves at these levels (the loop theory).
Some time later, Keegan and Garrett[45] reinvestigated the problem by
a method more similar to Head's than to that of Sherrington. The results
published by other investigators have not been essentially different from
those of Head or Sherrington.

Keegan and Garrett showed that in cases of disc protrusion it is very
unusual for more than one nerve root to be affected and that in cases
with compression of one nerve root an area of hypoalgesia can be marked
out in a repeatable fashion, even when conduction in the sensory fibres
has not been completely abolished. Their technique, briefly, was to use

a pin scratch of firmness adjusted to cause no more than a mildly unpleasant sensation in the hypoalgesic area. Using this method they found: '. . . that the dermatomes continue unbroken from dorsal midline to their termination in the limb, and that they have developed in a very different manner than postulated in the loop theory.' The charts which they drew are reproduced in Fig. 2.4.

During the course of the investigation, Keegan and Garrett found that they were able to map out, not only the main distribution of the nerve root but also a fainter overlap distribution extending often 2.5–5 cm (1–2 inches) on either side of the main distribution. It seems reasonable to think that the larger overlap distribution corresponds to Sherrington's area and the smaller to those outlined by Head. A comparison of the areas with those mapped by Head (Fig. 2.5) will show that in the distal part of the limb there is a very fair correspondence between the two. Fortunately, from the clinician's point of view, the proximal areas of the various dermatomes are of much less importance than the distal ones, about which there is fair general agreement.

When considering possible causes of pain in the buttock it is important to remember that the skin of the buttock is in part innervated by the cutaneous branches of the posterior primary division of the 11th and 12th thoracic nerves. This may be one mechanism by which pain in the buttock can be produced by problems in the low thoracic spine.

REFERENCES

 1. Mixter W. J., Barr J. S. (1934). Rupture of the intervertebral disc. *New Eng. J. Med;* **211**:210–215.
 2. Armstrong J. R. (1965). *Lumbar Disc Lesions,* 3rd edn. London: Livingstone.
 3. Brooke R. (1934). The sacro-iliac joint. *J. Anat;* **58**:299–305.
 4. Pitkin H. C., Pheasant H. C. (1936). Sacrarthrogenic telalgia. *J. Bone Jt Surg;* **18**:111–133, 365–374.
 5. Gray H. (1938). Sacro-iliac joint pain. *Int. Clin;* **2**:54–96.
 6. *Cunningham's Textbook of Anatomy,* 10th edn. (1964). London: Oxford University Press.
 7. Weisl H. (1955). Movement of the sacro-iliac joint. *Acta Anat;* **23**:80–91.
 8. *Gray's Anatomy, Descriptive and Applied,* 32nd edn. (1958). London: Longman.
 9. Fryette H. H. (1954). *The Principles of Osteopathic Technique.* Carmel: Academy of Applied Osteopathy.
10. Kapandji I. A. (1970). *The Physiology of the Joints,* Vol. 3, p. 70. London: Churchill Livingstone.
11. Schunke G. B. (1938). Anatomy and development of the sacro-iliac joint in men. *Anat. Rec;* **723**:313–331.
12. Kapandji I. A. (1970). *The Physiology of the Joints,* Vol. 3, p. 42. London: Churchill Livingstone.
13. Lovett R. W. (1900). The mechanics of lateral curvature of the spine. *Boston M.S.J;* **142**:622–627.
    Lovett R. W. (1902). The study of the mechanics of the spine. *Am. J. Anat;* **2**:457–462.

14. Schmincke A., Santo E. (1932). Zur normalen und pathologischen Anatomie der Halswirbelsaule. *Zbl. Path*; **55**:369–372.
15. Santo E. (1935). Zur Enwicklungsgeschichte und Histologie der Zwischenscheiben in den kleinen Gelenken. *Zeitschr. f. Anat. u. Entwicklungsgesch*; **104**:623–634.
16. Tondury G. (1940). Beitrag zur Kenntnis der kleinen Wirbelgelenke. *Zeitschr. f. Anat. u. Entwicklungsgesch*; **110**:568–575.
17. Zaccheo D., Reale E. (1955). Contributio alla cognoscenza delle articolazioni tra i processi articolari delle vertebre dell'uomo. *Archivio di Anatomia*; **61**:1–16.
18. Dorr W. M. (1958). Uber die Anatomie der Wirbelgelenke. *Arch. f. orthop. u. Unfall-Chir*; **50**:222–234.
19. Lewin T., Moffett B., Viidik A. (1961). The morphology of the lumbar synovial intervertebral joints. *Acta Morphologica Neerlando-Scandinavia*; **4**:299–319.
20. Hirsch C., Schajowicz F. (1952). Studies on structural change in the lumbar annulus fibrosus. *Acta orthopaed. Scand*; **22**:184–231.
21. Sylven B. (1951). On the biology of the nucleus pulposus. *Acta orthopaed. Scand*; **20**:275–279.
22. Hirsch C. (1959). Studies on the pathology of back pain. *J. Bone Jt Surg*; **41B**:237–247.
23. Lindblom K. (1951). Technique and results of disc puncture. *Acta orthopaed. Scand*; **20**:315–326.
24. Roofe P. G. (1939). Innervation of the annulus fibrosus. *Arch. Path*; **27**:201–211.
25. Werne S. (1959). The cranio-vertebral joints. *Acta orthopaed. Scand*; **28**:165–173.
26. Fielding J. W. (1957). Cineroentgenography of the normal cervical spine. *J. Bone Jt Surg*; **39A**:1280–1288.
27. Pedersen H. E., Blunk G. F. J., Gardner E. (1956). Anatomy of lumbo-sacral posterior rami. *J. Bone Jt Surg*; **38A**:377–391.
28. Wyke B. (1970). The neurological basis of thoracic spinal pain. *Rheumatol. Phys. Med*; **10**:356–366.
29. *Grant's Method of Anatomy*, 7th edn. (1965). Baltimore: Williams and Wilkins.
30. Penning L. (1968). *Functional Pathology of the Cervical Spine*. Amsterdam: Excerpta Medica.
31. Troup J. D. G. (1968). PhD thesis, London University.
32. Davis P. R. (1955). The thoraco-lumbar mortice joint. *J. Anat*; **89**:370–371.
33. Begg C., Falconer M. A. (1949). Plain radiography in intraspinal protrusions of intervertebral discs. *J. Bone Jt Surg*; **36**:225.
34. Froning E. C., Frohman B. (1968). Motion of the lumbo-sacral spine after laminectomy and spine fusion. *J. Bone Jt Surg*; **50A**:897–918.
35. Jirout J. (1955). Studies in the dynamics of the spine. *Excerpta Acta Radiol*; **46**: Fasc.
36. Bingham J. W. (1949). Some problems of causalgic pain. *Brit. Med. J*; **2**:334–338.
37. Barnes R. (1954). Causalgia in peripheral nerve injuries. *MRC Special Report Series 282*. London: HMSO.
38. Mitchell G. (1963). *The Anatomy of the Autonomic Nervous System*. Edinburgh: Livingstone.
39. Neuwirth E. (1960). Current concepts of the cervical portion of the sympathetic nervous system. *Lancet*; **80**:337–338.

40. Laruelle M. L. (1940). Les bases anatomique du systeme autonomic cortical et bulbo-spinal. *Rev. Neurol;* **72**:349–360.

41. Delmas J., Laux G., Guerrier Y. (1947). Comment atteindre les fibres pre-ganglionaires du membre superieur. *Gaz. Med. Fr;* **59**:703.

42. Tinel J. (1937). *Le Systeme Nerveux Vegetatif.* Paris: Masseon.

43. Head H. (1893). Disturbances of sensation with special reference to the pain of visceral disease. *Brain;* **16**:1–33, 339–480.

44. Sherrington C. S. (1893). Experiments in the examination of the peripheral distribution of the fibres of the posterior roots of some spinal nerves. *Phil. Trans;* **B184**:641–763; **B190**:45–187.

45. Keegan J. J., Garrett F. D. (1948). Segmental sensory nerve distribution. *Anat. Rec;* **102**:409–437.

Chapter 3

Examination, General Considerations, X-rays

In order to simplify description of examination techniques in this book the patient will be designated by the female gender and the examiner by the male.

THE SPINAL JOINT LESION

The characteristic signs of a spinal joint lesion for which manipulative treatment is likely to be appropriate are:

1. asymmetry,
2. restricted movement,
3. hypertonus in muscle and other soft tissues.

These three signs are entirely objective and must therefore be given more weight than the subjective sign of tenderness. It is usually possible to assess the likelihood of a subjective sign being of value in any particular patient. In those in whom these signs can be expected to be valuable, tenderness at the same level as the objective signs is useful confirmation of the presence of a joint lesion for which manipulation is likely to be helpful.

The acronym ART (asymmetry, restriction of motion, tension) or TART (tenderness ART) is useful as a reminder of the signs to be looked for.

There are often further signs which can be helpful by directing attention to a specific level. These are abnormalities of tissue texture, probably due to alteration of tone in the autonomic nerves to the part. These signs can be seen as a change in skin temperature locally, as a slight 'drag' when the hand is moved lightly across the skin at that level (due to increased moisture), as a resistance to 'skin rolling' or even as localised oedema. If the index and middle fingers are moved evenly down the paravertebral region with steady, moderate pressure, it will often be possible to see a 'red reaction', sometimes localised to one side. This can point to the need for detailed examination at that level.

Spinal joints when damaged have the property of losing part or all of their mobility. This, of course, also tends to happen to the more accessible joints, the more so if they are neglected after injury. As in the case of peripheral joints that have become stiff after injury, spinal joints with reduced mobility can remain symptomless for long periods. The precise reason why they should suddenly start to give trouble after remaining symptomless for such periods is still a matter for speculation. Experience strongly suggests that, with one exception, stiffened joints over which there is no detectable tissue tension abnormality are unlikely to be the source of major symptoms. The exception is the sacroiliac joint which is not closely bridged by its controlling muscles and any excess tension in them is not so easily felt by the examining finger.

It may not be possible to restore a full range of movement to a damaged joint. For the relief of symptoms, however, it is usually enough to restore some movement and to obtain correction of the tissue tension abnormality.

At this point it is appropriate to emphasise that this treatment is not dealing with dislocations, or subluxations, or a 'little bone out of place', nor is it putting back into place a 'slipped disc'. The diagnosis depends on the detection of motion restriction in a specific joint in at least one direction. The manipulation is designed to overcome this restriction specifically. X-rays are not of assistance in making this diagnosis. Although this principle is important, there are exceptions. There are some disturbances of pelvic function for which the term subluxation is correct, and which can be demonstrated by x-rays, but for which manipulation of this kind is the treatment of choice. Subluxation of the pubic symphysis is a common example.

The ability to detect tissue changes such as hypertonus, localised restriction of motion and subtle asymmetry requires training and improves greatly with practice and perseverance. Even the detection of skin drag is difficult at first. Some will have great difficulty to start with and many of us are not in the habit of using our hands as the sensitive tools that they are. The process can perhaps be compared to that of a novice trying to read Braille. Distinguishing the pattern of the raised dots is easy for those who have had sufficient practice. It is quite impossible for those, like one of the authors, who have not, and, to the beginner, the idea that it might be possible seems almost unbelievable. It is a good thing that there are many patients in whom the abnormalities of position, motion and tissue tension can be felt easily enough to convince all except the most bigoted disbelievers.

It may be as well to mention at this stage that the most common fault in learning this type of examination is the use of too much pressure. Gentle pressure allows one's proprioceptors to function much more efficiently.

THE BARRIER CONCEPT

A normal joint will move through a certain range of active motion. Beyond the end of what the muscles can do actively, there is a small additional passive range. From that point on, further movement can only occur if there is damage to ligament or bone and a fracture, dislocation or subluxation results. The barrier is the point at the end of the range and may be physiological (the end of the active movement), anatomical (the end of the passive range) or restrictive when for some reason there is partial loss of motion. This is illustrated by the diagrams in Fig. 3.1

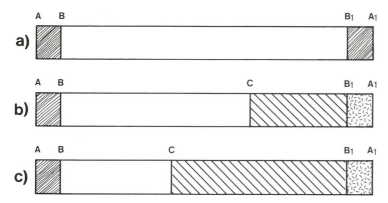

Fig. 3.1 The barrier concept. **(a)** Represents a normal joint. The range of physiological movement is represented as the distance between B and B₁. The total possible movement is that between A and A₁. The ranges A,B and A₁,B₁ are the passive ranges at either end. **(b)** Represents a joint with restricted motion. The available movement is now only from B to C with the passive range A,B. **(c)** Represents a major restriction, the remaining range being only about one-third of normal.

(after Kimberly[1]). Figure 3.1(a) is a diagram of a normal joint and the anatomical barrier is shown by A and A₁. The physiological barrier is shown at B and B₁.

In an abnormal joint of the kind that is under discussion there will be some alteration in movement, usually in the total range. Figure 3.1(b) is a diagram to show a relatively minor restriction of movement. There is now a new, restrictive barrier at C; motion is permitted between C and B (or A if passive motion is being considered). Figure 3.1(c) shows a more severe restriction with only a small amount of motion remaining. Patients are also seen in whom the range is limited in both directions. The barrier as shown in the diagram is, of course, in one plane only and for purposes of communication it is usual to describe barriers as they are found in the three cardinal planes of the standard anatomical position, sagittal or anteroposterior, coronal or right to left and transverse or horizontal.

It is very important to recognise that there will be a barrier in each of the three planes in almost all cases, and that, when it comes to treatment, it is vital to position the patient in such a manner that the barrier is engaged in all three planes.

The concept of a barrier to normal movement is of great importance because it is an objective sign which can be found and which can be felt to have changed after treatment. The object of treatment is to remove the barrier and there are a number of different ways in which this may be done. Two main methods will be described and the implications of the success of differing methods will be discussed.

At some point in the available range in every joint there will be a point of maximum ease. This is the point where the tissues around the joint are most relaxed, and movement in any direction will cause an increase in the tension of these tissues. In a normal joint this point is usually near the middle of the range but in a joint with an abnormal barrier it will probably move to near the midpoint of the remaining motion. It is possible to make use in treatment of the relaxation which will often occur when the joint is positioned so that it is kept at the point of maximum ease. This is a method of indirect treatment and techniques will not be described in this book, but the implications are important when one tries to find an explanation for what happens.

SOMATIC DYSFUNCTION

This term has now come into general use to describe the disturbance of joint function which was in the past known, among other names, as the osteopathic lesion. It is now the accepted term under which billing of medical insurers is accepted in the USA. It is defined as: 'Impaired or altered function of related components of the somatic (body framework) system; skeletal, arthrodial, and myofascial structures; and related vascular, lymphatic and neural elements.'

Other terms are used to describe the same process. The commonest are probably joint dysfunction and, in Europe, joint blockage. Both these suggest that the process is limited to the joint, which is probably not true. Regrettably 'subluxation' is still heard even with reference to spinal joints.

GENERAL EXAMINATION

Even in a practice that is entirely made up of patients referred by other physicians, it is important to recognise that the pain may be coming from other than a musculoskeletal source.

Pain in the upper chest on the left side may be due to somatic dysfunction in the low cervical or upper thoracic spine. It may also be due to coronary ischaemia and sometimes to both together. If the condition of the heart is known to be such that manipulative treatment is not contraindicated, it is recognised that removal of the part of the pain that is of musculoskeletal origin can be immensely helpful to a patient suffering from angina.

Abdominal pain may also arise either from a viscus or from disturbance of function in the appropriate region of the spine.

Low back pain may arise from a growth in the pelvis. It is always wise to do a rectal examination.

Herpes zoster often presents as a segmental pain and there will be tissue tension changes in the spinal tissues of that segment. It can be difficult to tell the difference in the early stages before the rash appears. Fortunately it does not appear to do any harm if one does make this mistake. One should always be gentle and the more so if the patient is in more than usual distress.

Anyone with a fairly acute viral infection is likely to have back pain and if patients develop such an infection during the course of treatment, it is wise to tell them to stay at home both for their own sakes and for those of your staff, your other patients and yourself! Treatment in these circumstances is unlikely to be very helpful anyway.

A careful neurological examination on the first visit is a wise precaution. In so many it will be normal, and if the only positive finding is a depressed or absent leg reflex, this is not a contraindication to treatment by manipulation, if this is otherwise appropriate. A repeat examination on future visits may be wise in order to assess progress and the more so in anyone who shows any sign of deterioration.

The dominant eye

When one is examining for small differences of level and rotation it is of great importance that one should have one's dominant eye over (or directly behind) the midline of the patient. If this is not done the effect of parallax will often be enough to mask the difference.

It can also be very helpful to get into the habit of using the response of one's proprioceptors, especially when estimating differences in level on the two sides. This can be most useful when examining the upper thoracic joints in a patient with medium or long hair. It is surprising how easily the art of feeling in this way can be learned.

To determine your dominant eye, make a circle with the index finger and thumb of one hand and hold it out in front at arm's length. With both eyes open, observe what is seen clearly through the circle. Then close each eye in turn. When the object originally seen remains in view, you are looking with your dominant eye. When the object changes, the dominant eye is the one that is closed.

THE MUSCULOSKELETAL SYSTEM

Referred pain is very common and, contrary to what many of us were taught, it often does not follow strictly in the expected pattern of dermatome, myotome or sclerotome. The work of Dr Janet Travell and Dr John Mennell on the pain patterns produced by myofascial trigger points does show that referred pain from these points is not always in segmental relation to the trigger point. Mennell[2] gives a series of diagrams which could with advantage be in the office of every physician practising in this field. He also describes one method of treatment for these pain-producing lesions. Travell and Simons[3] give an exhaustive account of trigger points above the diaphragm and the second volume of this very valuable text is in the late stages of preparation.

Because of paradoxical pain reference, it is not enough to assume that the dysfunction is at the level of the segmental nerve supply. Dr Philip Greenman puts it thus: 'It is no use chasing the pain'. What is required is a structural examination of the musculoskeletal system (and not just the spine!). If this is done it will sometimes be found that there are problems at a distance which, by mechanical or other means, upset the function of the symptomatic level.

Examination of every joint in the spine would take a very long time and even then there would be the limbs to look at. For this reason it is usual to divide the examination into an overall screen and a detailed examination of those areas to which one's attention is drawn in the screening, a process usually known as segmental definition. Some physicians insert a third stage which they call a scan. This is to refine the areas to be looked at in detail. When the segmental definition is completed it should be possible to pin-point the segment that requires attention and to know the position of the barrier in all three planes.

THE OVERALL SCREENING EXAMINATION

The influence of one part of the musculoskeletal system on the rest is such that abnormalities of structure in, for instance, the lower limbs can materially affect the spine. Simple dysfunction of limbs can also cause changes in spinal joint function. Problems in the upper limb usually have more effect on the upper half of the spine but lower limb dysfunction can be associated with spinal joint problems at any level.

Because of these connections, it is important that the screening examination should include both upper and lower limbs. Here again there is the question of the amount of time available. With practice it is possible to screen both upper and lower limbs in a very short time. The most important factors are asymmetries of size, muscle tension and range of motion between one side and the other. In the lower limb difference in length can be important.

STANDING EXAMINATION

1. Static, from behind.
(a) Compare the levels of:
    (i) the gluteal folds
    (ii) the trochanters
    (iii) the iliac crests
    (iv) the scapulae
    (v) the shoulders.
(b) Look for any tilting of the head.
(c) Rapidly scan the muscles of the feet, thighs and legs for differing tension.
(d) Is the gap between the elbow and trunk the same on the two sides? (Is there a scoliosis?)
2. Static, from the side.
(a) Is the 'gravity line' normal or is the head 'poked'?
(b) Are the spinal curves normal, exaggerated or flattened?
3. Static, from the front.
(a) Compare the height of the anterior superior iliac spines (ASISs) on each side.

(b) Compare the shoulder heights.

(c) Look for tilt of the head or rotation of the face.

4. With active movement. These tests are normally done from behind. The patient must be instructed to keep the knees straight.

(a) Note the range of flexion and of extension.

(b) Are there 'flat spots' where motion is restricted?

(c) Note restricted areas on sidebending to each side.

(d) Some operators may prefer the **hip drop test**. This is performed by having the patient allow one hip to drop by bending the knee on that side in order to sidebend the lumbar spine (Fig. 3.2). It is repeated for the other side.

5. A general test for function of the joints of the lower limb may be made by having the patient do a full knees bend with the feet flat on the floor. If this can be done, there is no major restriction. It is wise to instruct her to put a hand on the examination table for support.

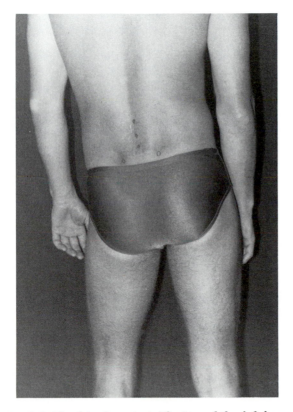

Fig. 3.2 The hip drop test. Flexion of the left knee allows the left side of the pelvis to drop, producing sidebending in the lumbar spine.

The standing forward flexion test

(Not a screening test but described here because it is performed with

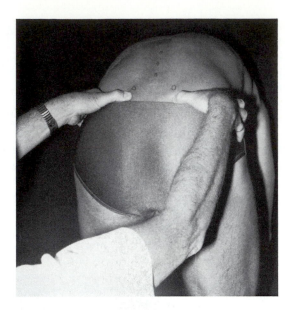

Fig. 3.3 Position at the end of the standing forward flexion test. The left thumb is slightly higher than the right, indicating stiffness of the left side of the pelvis.

the patient standing.) It is a test for loss of normal motion in the pelvis and does not provide a specific diagnosis, although it does indicate the side affected (Fig. 3.3).

1. The patient stands with the feet level but about 15 cm (6 inches) apart. The knees must be kept straight.

2. You stand or sit behind her.

3. Monitor the upward movement of the posterior superior iliac spines (PSISs) with your thumbs, which should be brought up from below to find the ledge under the PSIS on either side. This is the only point which is easy to compare.

4. Have the patient bend slowly forward while you observe which PSIS moves first and furthest.

5. **Note.**

(a) Unilateral hamstring tightness will give a false positive test. Test again after stretching.

(b) When the movement of the ilium on the sacrum is less on one side, the forward movement of the base of the sacrum will 'pick up' the ilium sooner on that side.

(c) *The side with restricted mobility is the one that moves first.*

SEATED EXAMINATION

There are five screening tests in this position.

1. Observe the relative heights of the PSIS. A different finding from

that in the standing examination suggests an anatomical difference in leg length.

2. Trunk rotation is tested actively by having the patient rotate her shoulders to the limit in each direction. A passive test may also be performed. The movement takes place primarily at the thoracolumbar junction and is normally about 90° to either side. The patient must be instructed to 'sit up tall' because slumping will restrict the range.

3. The function of the joints in the upper extremity can be assessed rapidly by having the patient raise her arms above her head with the backs of the hands together. If she can do this with the arms symmetrical about the head, function must be good.

4. Screening in the upper thoracic spine is most easily done by sidebending. The authors' preferred method is as follows (Fig. 3.4).

(a) The patient sits with her legs over the side of the examination table. It is important that she 'sits up tall'.

(b) You stand behind her.

(c) Place your right forearm across the patient's right shoulder, with your hand resting on the base of her neck.

(d) Your right index finger should point towards her left shoulder and your thumb points down her back. Your three remaining fingers curl round the base of her neck. Test by alternately pressing down on her right shoulder and then releasing and easing the trunk upright again.

(e) Monitor for movement at individual joints with your left thumb (or finger) at the side of each interspinous interval in turn.

(f) In the event of difficulty, the test may be repeated from the other side.

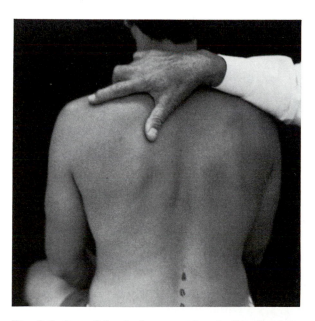

Fig. 3.4 A useful grip for screening in the thoracic spine.

5. Overall range in the cervical spine can be assessed. With the patient erect, the head should flex 45° on the neck and total flexion should be about 90°. Total extension is also about 90° in the normal. Normal sidebending is about 45°. Normal rotation is usually about 90° to each side.

SUPINE SCREENING

The screening examination is completed by testing rotation of the neck. The head is rolled, on the occiput, first to one side then to the other. If the chin can be brought to touch the shoulder on both sides without strain, the neck is considered to be fully mobile.

Examination in the supine position will be continued under the heading of detailed examination (Chapters 4 and 5).

The sitting forward flexion test (Fig. 3.5)

(This is not part of the overall screen but, as it and the flexed examination for lumbar rotation are most conveniently performed at this stage, they are described here.) It is similar to the standing test but, because the

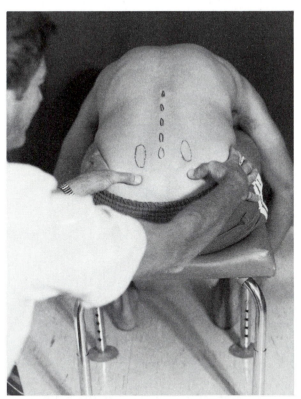

Fig. 3.5 Position at the end of the sitting forward flexion test. The right thumb is higher than the left, indicating stiffness of the right side of the pelvis.

weight is now on the ischial tuberosities instead of on the feet, the implications of a positive test are not quite the same.

1. The patient sits on a stool with her feet on the floor, or if she sits on a table, her feet must be supported to prevent her pitching forward.
2. She bends forward between her knees, as far as possible.
3. Again observe which PSIS rises first (and furthest).

Note. The sitting test is considered to indicate interference with pelvic motion from above because the effect of the legs is eliminated. The inference is that a positive sitting test indicates sacroiliac rather than iliosacral dysfunction. The distinction is not solely academic as it can lead to somewhat different treatment techniques.

EXAMINATION FOR ROTATION OF LUMBAR AND LOWER THORACIC VERTEBRAE IN FLEXION

This is conveniently done from the fully flexed, sitting position at the end of the sitting forward flexion test. If done standing, it leaves the patient in an uncomfortable position for longer than is necessary.

The test is performed by placing the thumbs over the back of each pair of transverse processes and observing any rotation as shown by the relative posteriority of the thumbs. It is often easier to see which thumb is the most posterior if one bends one's head and 'sights' along the thumbs.

ESTIMATION OF RELATIVE LEG LENGTH

The importance of a structural difference in the length of the legs is often overlooked. Even more common is failure to realise that estimation of relative leg length is difficult by any clinical test. The standard measurement from the anterior superior spine to the tip of the medial malleolus is open to gross errors if, as is so common, there is twisting of the pelvis. Measurement from the greater trochanter to the lateral malleolus is incomplete and tends to be inaccurate, especially in the obese. The clinical methods of estimation which are most helpful are as follows.

1. Comparison of the levels of the PSISs from behind with the patient standing. This is most easily done by finding the ledge under the PSIS from below with your thumbs and observing their relative heights with your dominant eye behind the patient's midline (Fig. 3.6).
2. Comparison of the heights of the PSISs from behind with the patient fully flexed so that you can 'sight along' the back and see which side is the higher (Fig. 3.7).
3. By observing the relative level of the gluteal folds from behind with the patient erect.
4. By comparing the relative height of the iliac crests with your index fingers placed horizontally along the crests (Fig. 3.8). Note that it is easy

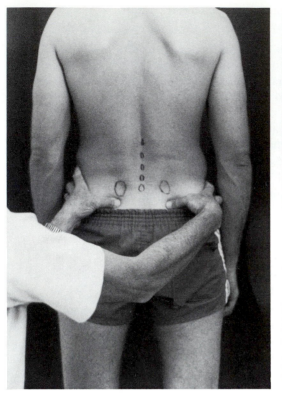

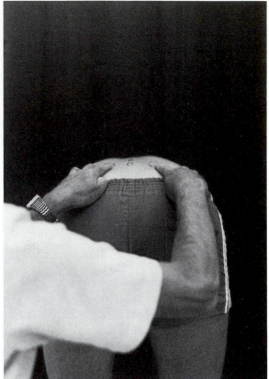

▲
Fig. 3.6 Examination for height of posterior iliac spines, standing.

▼
Fig. 3.7 Examination for height of posterior iliac spines in forward flexion, as a guide to relative leg length.

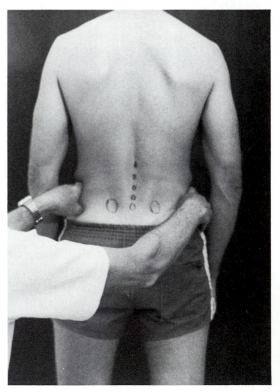

▶
Fig. 3.8 Examination for heights of iliac crests.

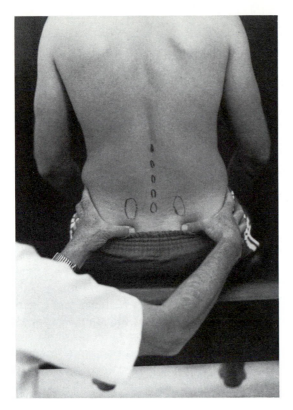

Fig. 3.9 Examination for relative heights of posterior spines, sitting.

to be misled by including a thicker layer of soft tissue on one side, the
more so in the presence of a scoliosis.

5. In some patients it is possible to distinguish between the short leg
and a twisted pelvis by examination from the front with the patient erect.
If the ASIS and the PSIS are higher on the same side, a difference in
leg length is indicated; if on opposite sides, the pelvis is probably twisted.

In all these examinations it is helpful to be aware of the information
given by one's proprioceptors as well as by one's eyes. The possibility
of observer error must always be remembered, even for those with long
experience.

If there is suspicion of a difference in leg length, you should next
examine the relative heights of the PSIS with the patient sitting (Fig.
3.9). With her sitting, the effect on PSIS height of leg length discrepancy
is eliminated.

1. If the right PSIS is lower than the left with the patient standing,
but level when she is sitting, there is evidence that the right leg is shorter
than the left.

2. If, with her sitting, the PSIS on the right still appears lower than
that on the left, the probable cause is a twisting of the pelvis with restriction of mobility.

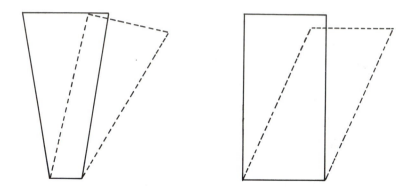

Fig. 3.10 Diagram to show the possible error in estimation of leg length if the feet are close together.

Dr James Fisk has pointed out that, in these estimations, an error can be introduced if the patient stands with her feet together. The error is relatively small unless there is marked unilateral spasm of the low lumbar or gluteal muscles. If, owing to such muscle spasm, the patient is leaning to one side, there will be a slight apparent increase in the length of the leg away from which she leans, because the feet are closer together than the hip joints. If the heels are placed about 15 cm (6 inches) apart, a parallelogram is formed, the base being the floor and the sides the lines joining the heels to the centre of movement of the hip joints. Simple geometry tells us that the relative heights of the hip joints must then remain the same even if the angle between the side and the base is changed (Fig. 3.10).

X-RAYS

If one is to rely on x-rays, it is of the utmost importance that the films are of good quality. Acceptance of evidence from poor quality films is dangerous. The beginner is very well advised to see recent x-ray pictures of every spine before he manipulates. With practice, he will find that his ability to assess the condition and the exact position of the vertebrae becomes good enough to justify confident diagnosis. Then, if techniques of the type described are used, without anaesthesia and without violence, a single manipulative treatment can be justified in many patients without the precaution of prior radiography.

If the result of such a manipulation is clearly beneficial, it is reasonable to postpone radiography until the improvement ceases or until some other cause makes it desirable. Indeed, it is often possible to treat a patient with somatic dysfunction without ever having x-rays. This practice is welcomed by many patients because of the present awareness of the dangers of radiation.

It is, of course, foolish to continue to treat anyone who has already had films taken without taking the trouble to see them. In this connection it is worth noting that, except for exclusion of some other pathology, films that are some months old will usually give almost all the information that one needs and repeat films are not often necessary.

Unfortunately, a negative x-ray is not proof of the absence of a variety of conditions that are better not manipulated. The manipulator must therefore maintain a high index of suspicion for a variety of contraindications. Of these, the most important are osteoporosis, infections and tumours.

Osteoporosis

Osteoporosis is only common in the comparatively elderly and is much more common in women. It is nearly always associated with loss of weight and will always show in an x-ray. If the spinal pain is due to osteoporosis, there has already been at least minor collapse of one or more vertebrae, even if this does not yet show in the x-rays. On the other hand, in many elderly patients with osteoporosis the pain is due to spinal joint dysfunction and will respond to gentle manipulation. In an elderly patient (and the more so if she has been losing weight) good x-rays should always be seen before manipulative treatment is started.

Infection

Infection is less important, being both less common and less likely to be missed on clinical grounds. The intensity and widespread nature of the muscle spasm over an infective lesion should immediately put the examiner on guard and remind him of its possible existence. The fact that the joint cannot be made to move at all by any technique for examination may also arouse his suspicion. The patient is usually ill. The patient with a straightforward back problem is in pain but not ill and the difference can be detected early in most instances. Fortunately the intensity of muscle spasm is sufficient for it to be unlikely that any harm will be done by a single manipulation of the type described in the following chapters, even in a patient with an early infective lesion.

Tumours

The same is not necessarily true of a tumour, and although the actual harm that can be done by a single manipulation of a joint in the neighbourhood of a tumour is probably small, this is a danger which must not be forgotten. It is important to remember that bone tumours do not always show in the x-rays, even when they are big enough to weaken the structure of the vertebral body.

Relative leg length

When x-ray pictures have been taken before the patient is seen for the first time, it is often sufficient to make use of them. If, however, radiogra-

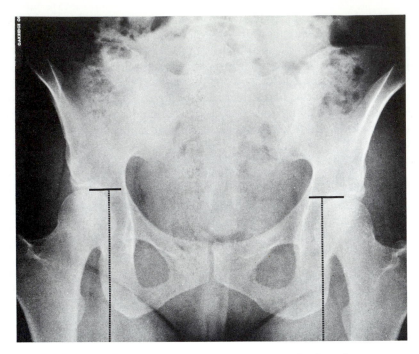

Fig. 3.11 X-ray showing a structural difference in leg length.

phy is being undertaken for the purpose, certain special views can be obtained which are of assistance. In the lumbar region it is always desirable to have the standard AP and lateral pictures with obliques to show the integrity of the pedicles and the condition of the facet joints. An anteroposterior picture of the pelvis taken with the patient standing erect, heels on the ground and knees straight, is of great value in assessing any difference in the actual length of the legs (Fig. 3.11).

For the examination to be accurate, care must be taken to ensure that the edge of the cassette lies parallel to the floor, or, because that is difficult, to incorporate a marker on the film. This has often been done by a radio-opaque plumb line suspended in front of the film. A simpler and more accurate method, which does not suffer from the disadvantage of the plumb line which must be allowed to hang free, has been devised by Dr Colin Harrison of Vancouver.

Dr Harrison's method is to use a closed hoop of plastic tubing about 22.5 cm (9 inches) in diameter, half-filled with a radio-opaque fluid. The hoop is attached by adhesive tape to the x-ray table in such a position that the fluid meniscus on either side is somewhere near the level of the hip joints (Fig. 3.12). A pencil line on the film joining the shadow of the two menisci gives an accurate level. From this line any difference in the height of the hip joints can be measured with a ruler and simple subtraction. Other methods of measuring the length of the legs by x-rays are available and are probably more accurate. However, this method has the advantage of simplicity and of providing a 'functional' picture of the pelvis, that is to say, one taken during weightbearing.

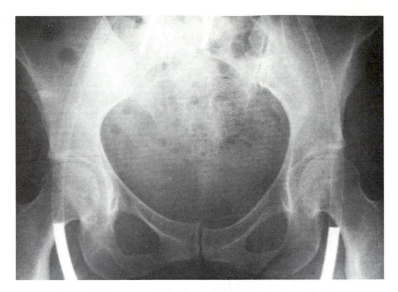

Fig. 3.12 A method of x-ray measurement of relative leg length. The patient is standing in a precise position. The marker is a plastic tube half-filled with radio-opaque fluid.

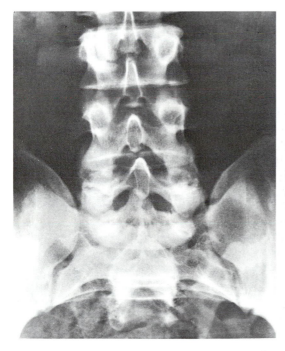

Fig. 3.13 Deviation of spinous process of L4 to the left side.

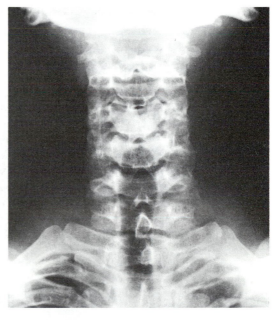

Fig. 3.14 Deviation of spinous process of T1 to the right side.

The 'erect pelvis' film will show the difference in actual leg length and it will also show if there is significant tilt of the sacral base, which is the parameter preferred by Greenman.[4]

Vertebral rotation

When examining an AP film, it is of interest to note any deviation from the midline of the spinous process of a single vertebra (Figs. 3.13 and 3.14). Of more importance is the finding of a different distance of the spinous process from the pedicle on one side than on the other. If there is a general deviation of a group of processes in one region, it indicates a type I lesion, that is, a lesion of the type that occurs in neutral flexion/ extension, where vertebral rotation is to the convexity of the sidebend curve. The finding of a spinous process deviated to the convexity of a short lateral curve (i.e. with the body rotated to the concavity) indicates a type II lesion occurring in either flexion or extension. These lesions are nearly always caused by trauma and should be treated first. It must be remembered that in the cervical spine above C7, the spinous processes are not usually symmetrical. Assessment of rotation by spinous process position is not reliable above C7 or, occasionally, C6.

Radiological demonstration of loss of mobility

A technique for showing sacroiliac mobility by x-rays was devised by Chamberlain.[5] The authors do not use this method but it could provide a convincing demonstration of sacroiliac mobility for those who still doubt.

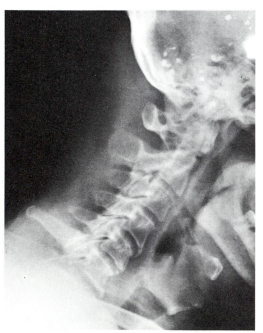
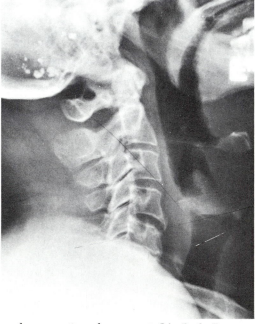

a   b

Fig. 3.15 Cervical spine showing degenerative changes at C4, 5, 6, 7; comparison of flexion (a) and extension (b) views shows immobility of C2–3 as well as generalised diminished movement.

Lumbar stiffness can be seen if lateral films are taken in flexion and extension, but the information is of little extra value and probably does not justify the extra radiation.

In addition to the standard projection for the cervical spine, lateral pictures taken in three additional positions may be helpful. They involve

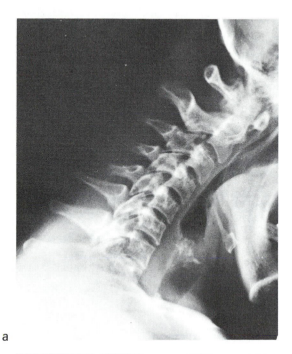

a

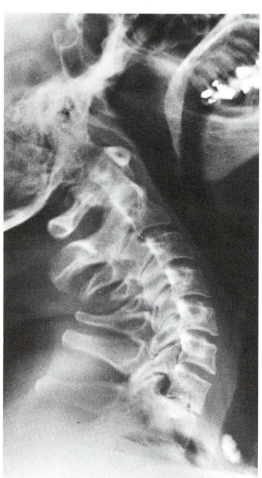

b

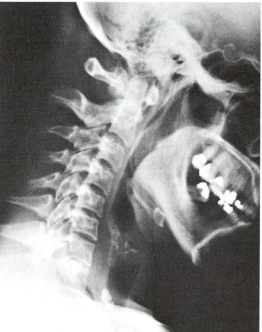

Fig. 3.16 The three lateral x-ray views of the cervical spine. There is diminished mobility at the atlanto-occipital joint: **(a)** full flexion, **(b)** full extension, and **(c)** head flexion ('chin tucked in').

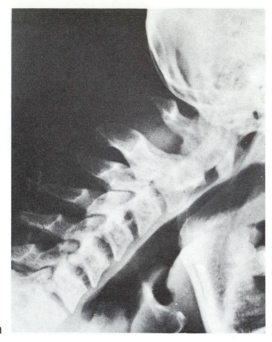

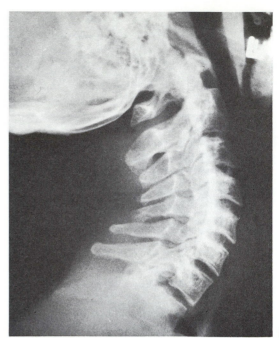

Fig. 3.17 Three lateral views demonstrating mobility at the atlanto-occipital joints: **(a)** full flexion, **(b)** full extension (note absence of demonstrable movement at C0–1), **(c)** head flexion showing opening of gap between occiput and arch of atlas.

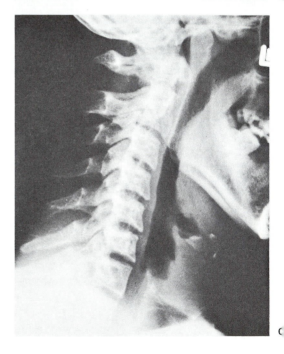

greater exposure and their value must be considered in this light, but if they are taken the standard lateral can be omitted. The three positions are full flexion, full extension and full flexion of the head on the neck with no flexion of the lower neck joints. This is obtained by asking the patient to 'tuck the chin well in'.

From a comparison of the flexed and extended films, the range of movement of the intervertebral joints can be measured (Fig. 3.15). The additional film with the chin tucked in is required for assessment of movement at the atlanto-occipital joint (Figs. 3.16 and 3.17). In full flexion of the neck there tends to be some unfolding of the head, in order to get the chin out of the way, and therefore the occipitoatlantal joint is not in full flexion. This joint may appear not to move when the full flexion film is compared with that in full extension, but its mobility may still be demonstrated by the third film. Details of techniques for estimating the actual movement at the individual joints are given by Penning.[6]

REFERENCES

1. Kimberly P. E. (1980). Formulating a prescription for osteopathic manipulative treatment. *JAOA*; **79**:506–513.
2. Mennell J. M. (1975). The therapeutic use of cold. *JAOA*; **74**:1146–1158.
3. Travell J. G., Simons D. G. (1983). *Myofascial Pain and Dysfunction*. Baltimore: Williams and Wilkins.
4. Greenman P. E. (1978). Lift therapy: use and abuse. *JAOA*; **79**:238–250.
5. Chamberlain W. E. (1932). The X-ray examination of the sacro-iliac joint. *Delaware State Med J*; **4**:195–201.
6. Penning L. (1968). *Functional Pathology of the Cervical Spine*. Amsterdam: Excerpta Medica.

Chapter 4

Detailed Examination:
The Pelvis

Nomenclature

There is a troublesome diversity of names for many of the dysfunctions in the pelvic ring. Members of the osteopathic profession are the ones who have worked out the details in greater depth than anyone else and, although even they use different names among themselves, the nomenclature in this edition has been brought more into line with the mainstream of osteopathic thought. In particular, the distinction of iliosacral and sacroiliac which has already been mentioned. This distinction helps in the understanding of both diagnostic and treatment procedures.

The names used for the various pelvic dysfunctions are those most recently agreed upon and for which changes were necessary. One movement of the sacrum was variously known by one group as flexion and by another group (in a slightly different context) as extension!

In order to avoid ambiguity, it may be as well to record that the term **sulcus** is used here to refer to the interval between the PSIS and the back of the sacrum unless otherwise specifically stated.

Anatomy

The pelvis is a three part bony ring consisting of the two innominate bones (which are properly regarded as part of the lower limbs) and the sacrum, which is formed of five vertebrae fused together and which, in some ways behaves as an atypical lumbar vertebra.

If it were a simple mechanical model, it would not matter whether we looked at the pelvis from the point of view of the innominates moving on the sacrum, or from that of the sacrum moving between the innominates. In the living body, however, the position is complicated by weight-bearing and by the action of muscles both in the trunk and the legs. This muscle action is more important when it is disordered, as it so often is in patients with back and leg symptoms.

When the patient is standing erect, the pelvis is influenced by both structural and functional asymmetry of the lower limbs. (The position adopted by the pelvis to accommodate for leg length discrepancy has been discussed in Chapter 2.) Imbalance of length or strength of lower limb muscles also produces a disturbance of function in the pelvic joints.

When the patient is seated, the innominates are stabilised by the weight being borne on the ischial tuberosities, and the precise position of the sacroiliac joints is then much more influenced by the position of the spine and the tension in the trunk muscles. Similarly, if the patient lies prone, the pelvis is supported by the pubes and the anterior superior spines, leaving the sacrum to respond to the influence of the trunk. On the other hand, in the supine position, the sacrum is stabilised by weight-bearing on the table and the innominates are then responding to tensions from below.

Because of this functional difference, the concept has developed that there is a difference between iliosacral dysfunction (that of the innominate on the sacrum) and sacroiliac dysfunction (that of the sacrum between the innominates). This concept is found to be helpful in some clinical situations but there are experienced manipulators who do not make the distinction.

The diagnostic method to be described will incorporate this distinction but, for those who wish to use the simpler approach, the parts that can be omitted will be indicated.

Landmarks

In making a diagnosis of pelvic dysfunction, the most important landmarks are as follows.

1. The anterior superior iliac spines (ASIS) for relative height and anteriority.
2. The superior pubic rami, or tubercles, for relative height.

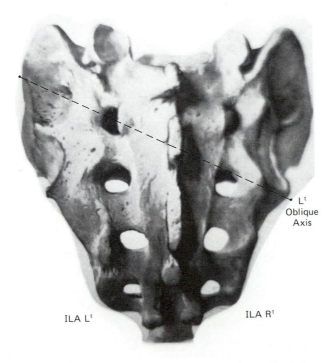

L¹
Oblique
Axis

ILA L¹   ILA R¹

Fig. 4.1 Posterior view of sacrum to show the left oblique 'axis' and the inferior lateral angles (ILA).

3. The posterior superior iliac spines (PSIS) for relative height and posteriority.

4. The apparent relative leg length as shown by the levels of the medial malleoli, both prone and supine.

5. The sacral base for rotation. This is felt in the sulcus between the PSIS and the spines of S1 and S2. The position of the sacral base is not necessarily indicated by the depth of the sacral sulcus. That may be a useful pointer but is also affected by the innominate position.

6. The inferior lateral angles (ILAs) of the sacrum for posteriority and inferiority. These are found about 1.9 cm (0.75 inch) from the midline, at the level of the sacral hiatus (Fig. 4.1).

7. The ischial tuberosities for relative height.

8. The sacrotuberous ligaments for relative tightness.

Sacral motion

The possible movements of the sacrum are as follows.

1. Anterior and posterior nutation (movement respectively forward and downward or backward and upward of the sacral base). This is sometimes known as flexion or extension, respectively. As the sacrum bends forwards it also slides down the auricular surface of the ilium so that the movement is not a simple rotation about an axis.

2. Anterior or forward torsion. In torsion the sacrum rotates about a theoretical oblique axis running from the superior pole of the sacroiliac joint on one side to the opposite inferior pole. The axis takes its name from the side of the superior pole. Rotation of the sacrum and vertebrae is named by the side to which the anterior aspect of the bone turns. Anterior torsion is when the sacrum turns toward the side of the axis. This rotation is accompanied by sidebending to the opposite side. Anterior torsion on the left oblique axis involves turning of the sacrum so that the front faces toward the left. For brevity this is often referred to as **left on left torsion.** Anterior torsion is a normal physiological movement and occurs in normal walking. Symptoms arise only when the mechanism becomes stiffened in this position.

3. Posterior or backward torsion. The sacrum can also rotate to the side opposite to the axis. This is posterior torsion. It is not a physiological movement and is almost always caused by trauma. It is frequently the source of relatively severe symptoms and is rarely an isolated lesion. Other pelvic dysfunctions with or without lumbar lesions are the rule rather than the exception. It is one of the causes of the 'well man bends over, cripple stands up' syndrome. Posterior sacral torsion to the right on the left oblique axis is associated with sidebending of the sacrum to the left.

Innominate motion

The normal movements of the innominates are antagonistic rotations about a transverse axis through the symphysis pubis. These can only take place at the same time as the physiological torsion of the sacrum. Examination of a pelvis will quickly show that such rotation is essential in order to allow torsion. Again, symptoms only arise when the mechanism loses its mobility and this can happen at either end of the range. There are also abnormal, unphysiological movements of the innominates which may properly be termed subluxations.

1. Physiological movements.

(a) Posterior rotation of one innominate on the sacrum. This is usually known as the posterior innominate, occasionally as the anterior sacrum. This movement cannot occur without the opposite movement on the other side. The lesion takes its name from the side that has restricted mobility.

(b) Anterior rotation of one innominate: anterior innominate (or posterior sacrum).

2. Unphysiological movements. These can only take place if the shape of the sacroiliac joint surfaces is unusual. For the shears, there must be an absence of the change in joint bevel usually found at about the S2 segment. For the flares, the joint surfaces must be rounded from before backward in order to allow rotation of the ilium about an axis parallel to the long axis of the sacrum. Such variations in sacroiliac joint shape are uncommon but not rare.

(a) Superior innominate shear (upslip). This is the most important. It is uncommon but not rare and is one of the causes of the 'failed back'. The innominate slides up on the sacrum and it may be produced by a fall on one buttock, by repeatedly stepping down from a height with the leg straight, as do some truck drivers, or even by missing a step. It is usually associated with other lesions in the pelvis or lumbar spine.

(b) Inferior innominate shear (downslip). This is rare and will usually be self-correcting on weightbearing. It is probably produced by falling forward with the foot caught.

(c) Inflare and outflare lesions are rare. The ASIS will be found to be further in for the former, or further out for the latter than its fellow. The abnormal side will be indicated by the positive standing forward flexion test.

Pubic motion

Normal motion at the pubic symphysis is rotation about a transverse axis only. Abnormal movement can occur and is properly called **subluxation**; when present it interferes with the normal rotation. Because rotation is an essential part of the physiological motion of the pelvis in walking, examination and treatment for pubic dysfunction are considered the first priority.

The abnormal movements are as follows.

1. A 'vertical' shear. The pubis on one side, at the symphysis, is higher than on the other. This is palpable and can be seen on x-ray (Fig. 4.2). On the abnormal side there is sometimes tenderness and tightness in the tissues at the pubic tubercle, at the insertion of the inguinal ligament.

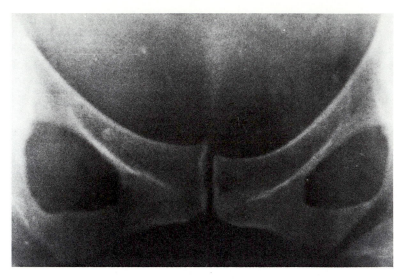

Fig. 4.2 Pubic symphysis showing subluxation.

The standing forward flexion test will usually be positive on the abnormal side.

2. A simple separation. This is much less common but can also be felt and seen on x-ray.

3. An anteroposterior displacement. Uncommon and usually slight.

DETAILED EXAMINATION

1. Standing.
(a) The levels of PSISs.
(b) The levels of ASISs.
(c) The standing forward flexion test (standing FFT).
(d) The levels of the superior pubic rami. (Usually examined with the patient supine.)

2. Sitting.
(a) The sitting forward flexion test (sitting or seated FFT).
(b) With the patient flexed, rotation of lumbar vertebrae as shown by the position of the transverse processes.
(c) The position of the ILAs on forward flexion. Look for any change in posteriority or inferiority.

3. Supine.
(a) The levels of the pubic rami, or tubercles. Note any tissue texture change at either pubic tubercle. If this test is positive, that is, if the levels are unequal, *stop*. Treat the pubic dysfunction and then start the examination again at the standing FFT.
(b) In case of doubt as to which side is abnormal, the pubic ramus on one side (and then on the other) can be moved up and down between the index finger and the thumb. It is important that one should not grip

the ramus tightly because that is painful. The movement is small. The side that moves less well is the side to treat.

(c) The relative heights of the iliac crests. If there is a difference, suspect an innominate shear: *stop*. Check for this and, if it is present, treat it before proceeding.

(d) The position of the ASISs with respect to relative height, anteriority and distance from the midline.

(e) The relative height of the medial malleoli which, in this position, is a function of innominate rotation unless there is a structural difference in the length of the legs.

4. Prone.

(a) The relative heights and posteriority of the PSISs.

(b) The position of the sacral base in the horizontal plane: is one side more posterior than the other? (See note.)

(c) The ILA position with respect to the relative posteriority or inferiority on the two sides.

(d) The depth of the lumbar lordosis or the spring test. The spring test is performed by pressing down on the lumbar spine with one or both hands. The arms should be straight for better control. A resistance to simple springing indicates a positive test and signifies a flattened lordosis.

(e) The relative heights of the ischial tuberosities. To be significant there should be a difference of at least 7 mm (0.25 inch).

(f) The relative tightness of the sacrotuberous ligaments.

(g) The relative leg length as shown by the height of the medial malleoli with the feet over the end of the table. In this position, if the legs are structurally equal, a difference is likely to be due to a lumbar scoliosis.

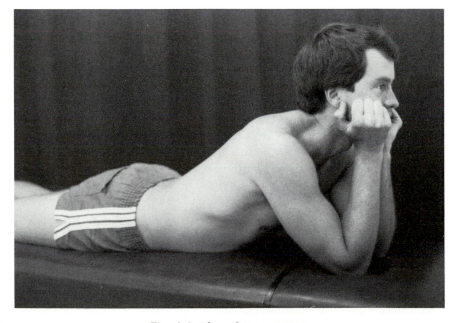

Fig. 4.3 The sphinx position.

(h) The rotation of one or more of the lumbar vertebrae as shown by the transverse process position, now in the neutral position.

5. Prone in hyperextension, the **sphinx position**. The patient hyperextends her spine by bringing her elbows close together at the level of the neck, supporting her head in her hands as high as she can and allowing her abdominal wall to relax (Fig. 4.3).

(a) The ILA position for exaggeration or lessening of asymmetry.

(b) The sacral base position for exaggeration or lessening of asymmetry.

(c) The rotation of lumbar vertebrae in extension.

Notes

1. In the forward flexion tests, the sooner the innominate moves the worse is the restriction of movement. *The PSIS which moves first and further in a vertical direction is on the side with limited movement, i.e. of the positive test.*

2. If the FFT is more strongly positive standing than sitting, suspect that the cause is iliosacral or pubic or from below. If the sitting test is the worse, suspect sacroiliac dysfunction.

3. When estimating the sacral base position, press in for a few moments with a finger on each side to disperse the fluid which is often there and which may give a false impression.

4. In any sacral dysfunction, look for maladaptive lumbar lesions and, if present, treat them before final assessment of the sacrum. This is especially important with a posterior torsion when there is nearly always one or more type II lumbar lesions.

5. Pelvic dysfunctions are commonly multiple.

6. In recurrent iliosacral lesions, always check the legs.

DIAGNOSIS

Simpler approach

This method of making the diagnosis in pelvic dysfunction will work well with a majority of patients. The actual treatment of the pelvis itself is limited to that of distortion of the pubic symphysis and the correction of innominate dysfunction. The latter is itself limited to the problems of the anterior and posterior innominate.

The success of this method in treatment of some of the pelvic dysfunctions appears to result from the reaction of the sacrum to correction of dysfunction in the lumbar spine. If the lumbar spine is treated first, it will often be found that the sacroiliac (as distinct from iliosacral) dysfunctions will be corrected by treating them as if they were indeed iliosacral.

Consideration of the anatomy will show that, for instance, the common anterior sacral torsion on the left oblique axis must be associated with a posterior position of the right innominate and an anterior position of that on the left. It is not necessarily clear on which side the restriction of movement will be found.

In general, a posterior innominate is a more frequent cause of symptoms than an anterior one, although, if restricted, the anterior can also require treatment. As will be shown in the section on diagnosis of torsions (see p. 66), it is usual to find that, in an anterior torsion, the sitting forward flexion test is positive on the side opposite the axis. This suggests that in a patient with a left anterior sacral torsion, the main restriction of sacroiliac motion is on the right side and, if this is what is found, the appropriate treatment would be that of a right posterior innominate—after the lumbar spine had been treated.

Even if one decides to adopt the simpler approach, the superior innominate shear may occasionally cause a problem. The treatment of this is relatively simple and it is of interest to note that the same manoeuvre was at one time described as a treatment for the posterior innominate. It may be that this technique should be added to those listed.

For the simpler approach, the diagnostic tests are all described in the fully specific section and will simply be listed here. Other tests can be added if desired.

1. Standing forward flexion test.
2. Sitting forward flexion test. Useful especially if the patient is unable to bend forward while standing. In this position one should also assess the lumbar vertebrae for rotation.
3. The heights of the superior pubic rami.
4. Tissue texture abnormality (TTA) at the pubic tubercle.
5. The relative height and anteriority of the ASISs.
6. The relative height and posteriority of the PSISs. With the patient prone for this examination, the lumbar vertebral rotations can be assessed both in neutral and in extension.
7. TTA in the sulcus between the PSIS and the sacrum.
8. A further test for restriction of movement in the sacroiliac joint if desired.

Fully specific approach

The different varieties of pelvic dysfunction to be considered are as follows.

1. Pubis.
(a) Superior subluxation at the symphysis.
(b) Inferior subluxation at the symphysis.
(c) Separation at the symphysis.
2. Sacroiliac.
(a) Anterior, or forward, sacral torsion. Left on left or right on right. Left is very common, right less common.
(b) Posterior, or backward, sacral torsion. Right on left or left on right. Both are uncommon but not rare. Always traumatic in origin. These are frequently associated with other dysfunctions in the pelvic mechanism and often produce severe symptoms.

(c) Inferior sacral shear. (Formerly called unilateral sacral flexion.) Common on the left side, rare on the right; may be bilateral.

(d) Superior sacral shear. (Formerly called unilateral sacral extension.) Much less common than the inferior shear and found more often on the right side. May be bilateral. Usually the result of trauma and may be found in those injured in rear-end collisions.

3. Iliosacral.

(a) Anterior innominate. More common on the right than the left.

(b) Posterior innominate. More common on the left.

(c) Superior innominate shear (upslip). Uncommon but important; more common on the left than on the right.

(d) Inferior innominate shear (downslip). Rare.

(e) Outflare. Uncommon; can only occur with an unusual sacral shape.

(f) Inflare. Uncommon; as outflare.

Diagnostic findings

The findings will be described for one side only because, in each case, the findings will be the same on the other side, if the side labels are reversed.

Note that the only difference in findings between an anterior and a posterior torsion is in the state of the lumbar lordosis. If there is doubt about the lordosis, the springing test may be used or the change in signs when the patient moves from flexion of the lumbar spine into the sphinx or extended position.

1. Superior pubis on the right.

(a) Standing forward flexion test, positive right.

(b) Pubic tubercle and superior ramus, high right.

(c) Inguinal ligament, tender and tense right.

(d) The right pubis does not move easily on direct motion testing.

2. Inferior pubis on the left.

(a) Standing flexion test, positive left.

(b) Pubic tubercle, low left (high right).

(c) Inguinal ligament, tender and tense left.

(d) The left pubis does not move easily on direct motion testing.

3. Separated symphysis. A gap may be felt, the tubercles will be level and the forward flexion tests may be negative.

4. Anterior or forward torsion, left on left oblique axis.

(a) Sitting flexion test, positive right.

(b) Sitting ILA test, positive left (the asymmetry is exaggerated on flexion).

(c) Inferior lateral angle, posterior and slightly inferior left, more so on flexion. May become level in extension.

(d) Base of sacrum, anterior right.

(e) Lumbar lordosis, increased and signs reduced by extension of the spine. Springing test negative.

(f) Lumbar scoliosis, convex right.

(g) Medial malleolus, prone, high left.

(h) Lumbar adaptation, L5 rotated right.

5. Posterior or backward torsion, right on left oblique axis.

(a) Sitting flexion test, positive right.

(b) Sitting ILA test, negative.

(c) Inferior lateral angle, posterior and slightly inferior right, more so in extension. May become level in flexion.

(d) Base of sacrum, posterior right.

(e) Lumbar lordosis, reduced and signs worse in extension of the spine. Springing test positive.

(f) Lumbar scoliosis, convex left.

(g) Medial malleolus, prone, high right.

(h) Lumbar adaptation, L5 rotated left.

6. Unilateral inferior sacral shear, left (formerly known as unilateral sacral flexion).

(a) Sitting flexion test, positive left.

(b) Inferior lateral angle, inferior, and slightly posterior left. Never becomes level on flexion or extension.

(c) Base of sacrum, anterior left.

(d) Lumbar lordosis, normal or increased.

(e) Lumbar scoliosis, convex left.

(f) Medial malleolus, prone, low left.

(g) Lumbar adaptation, right sidebending.

7. Unilateral superior sacral shear, right (formerly known as unilateral sacral extension).

(a) Sitting flexion test, positive right.

(b) Inferior lateral angle, superior right, and slightly anterior. Never becomes level on flexion or extension.

(c) Base of sacrum, posterior right.

(d) Lumbar lordosis, reduced.

(e) Lumbar scoliosis, convex left.

(f) Medial malleolus, high right.

(g) Lumbar adaptation, right sidebending.

8. Bilateral sacral shears.

(a) Sitting flexion test, positive on both sides. Both innominates start to move immediately.

(b) Lumbar lordosis, increased in inferior shears, reduced in superior shears.

(c) The other signs are negative, being the same on each side.

9. Anterior innominate right.

(a) Standing flexion test, positive right.

(b) ASIS supine, inferior right.

(c) Medial malleolus supine, low right.

(d) PSIS prone, superior right.

(e) Sacral sulcus prone, shallow right.

10. Posterior innominate left.

(a) Standing flexion test, positive left.

(b) ASIS supine, superior left.

(c) Medial malleolus supine, high left.

(d) PSIS prone, inferior left.

(e) Sacral sulcus prone, deep left.

11. Superior innominate shear (upslip) left.

(a) Standing flexion test, positive left.

(b) Iliac crest, superior left, prone and supine.

(c) Medial malleolus, high left, prone and supine.

(d) PSIS prone, superior left.

(e) Ischial tuberosity prone, superior left.

(f) Sacrotuberous ligament prone, lax left.

12. Inferior innominate shear right.

(a) Standing flexion test, positive right.

(b) Iliac crest, inferior right, prone and supine.

(c) Medial malleolus, low right, prone and supine.

(d) PSIS prone, inferior right.

(e) Ischial tuberosity prone, inferior right.

(f) Sacrotuberous ligament prone, tight right.

13. Inflare right.

(a) Standing flexion test, positive right.

(b) ASIS supine, medial right.

(c) PSIS prone, lateral right.

(d) Sacral sulcus prone, wide right.

14. Outflare left.

(a) Standing flexion test, positive left.

(b) ASIS supine, lateral left.

(c) PSIS prone, medial left.

(d) Sacral sulcus prone, narrow left.

It will be seen from the above that the signs of, for instance, an anterior innominate on the right are similar to those of a posterior innominate on the left. The major difference is in the side of the positive flexion test. Sometimes, even when it is clear that there is restriction of pelvic motion, it may be difficult to interpret the findings of the flexion tests. In such a patient it is helpful to use one, or more, of the other tests for sacroiliac mobility . The authors' preference is for the prone springing test.

ADDITIONAL TESTS FOR SACROILIAC MOBILITY

1. The prone springing test (Fig. 4.4).

(a) The patient lies prone.

(b) To test the right sacroiliac joint you stand to her right and place two fingers of your right hand so that the tips rest on the sacral base and the front of the terminal phalanx is in contact with the medial aspect of the PSIS.

(c) Use the heel of your left hand to spring the right side of the apex of the sacrum. This is most easily done with the left elbow straight. The range of movement is small but it is usually possible to feel the difference between a mobile and an immobile joint.

2. The supine springing test (Fig. 4.5).

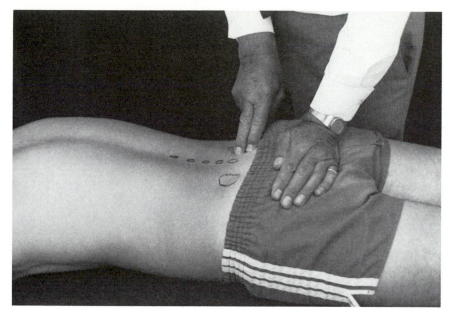

Fig. 4.4 The prone springing test for sacroiliac mobility.

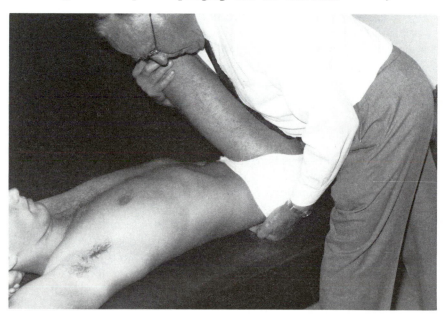

Fig. 4.5 The supine springing test for sacroiliac mobility.

(a) The patient lies supine.

(b) To test the right sacroiliac joint you stand to her right.

(c) Flex her right hip and knee fully and control the limb by holding it in your right axilla and with your right hand.

(d) Slide your left hand under her right buttock until your fingertips can palpate the sulcus between the PSIS and the sacrum.

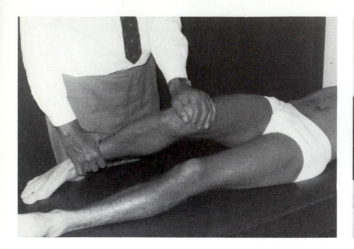

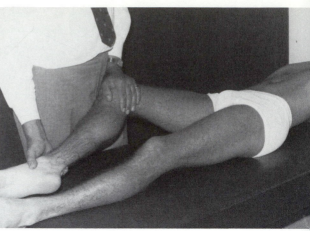

Fig. 4.6 Test for sacroiliac motion. Position at the end of the leg-shortening manoeuvre.

Fig. 4.7 Test for sacroiliac motion. Position at the end of the leg-lengthening manoeuvre.

(e) Lock her right femur against the ilium by full flexion and adduction. If necessary, the stability of the left side of the pelvis can be increased by allowing the left leg to drop over the side of the table.

(f) Rock the ilium on the sacrum by alternately increasing and decreasing the adduction and flexion of the thigh while you monitor for motion at the joint with your left hand.

3. The leg lengthening test (Figs. 4.6 and 4.7).

(a) The patient lies supine.

(b) In order to remove any chance asymmetry, ask her to put her feet flat on the table; lift her pelvis and then put it down again.

(c) Ask her to extend her legs on the table and note the relative levels of the medial malleoli.

(d) With the patient relaxed, you pick up each of her legs in turn and put each through similar movements, afterwards returning the leg to the table beside its fellow. After each movement you check the levels of the medial malleoli.

(e) To shorten the leg (if the sacroiliac joint is mobile), flex the knee and hip in abduction and external rotation to full flexion in neutral and then through adduction and internal rotation back to the table.

(f) To lengthen the leg (if the sacroiliac joint is mobile), flex the knee and hip in adduction and internal rotation to full flexion in neutral and then back to the table through abduction in external rotation. The difference in height of the medial malleoli in normal mobility is about 13 mm (0.5 inch) on each side. The mechanism by which this alteration of apparent leg length is produced was described in Chapter 2 (see Fig. 2.2).

Tenderness and muscle hypertonus around the sacroiliac joint

Tenderness in muscle on the lateral aspect of the ilium is very common in low back problems. Often it is possible to find areas of localised hypertonus and these may sometimes be true Travell trigger points. That for the gluteus medius is found below the iliac crest, a short distance lateral to the PSIS, and that for the minimus more laterally, near the mid-lateral line.

If true Travell triggers are present, they should be treated by cold spray and stretching or injection of the trigger point with local anaesthetic (plain and *no* steroid) followed by stretching. It is common to find areas of tender hypertonic muscle that do not fit the true trigger point description. These often disappear when the, apparently causative, spinal lesion has been successfully treated. If they persist, they may also be treated in a similar manner. There is sometimes evidence to suggest that these areas can, if persistent, cause the spinal lesion to recur.

There are three points close to the sacroiliac joint which deserve special mention.

1. The first is over the sacral base between the PSIS and the spinous processes of S1 and 2 (Fig. 4.8, 1). This is tender in many patients who have dysfunction at the sacroiliac joint. It does not give any indication of the nature of the dysfunction and, indeed, the restriction of motion is often on the other side.

2. The second is a little higher, between the PSIS and the spinous process of L5 (Fig. 4.8, 2). This is the typical point at which tenderness is found in problems at the lumbosacral joint. It must be remembered, however, that this tenderness is not of itself enough to make that diagnosis. Many patients who have had back surgery, and a number who have not, will be found to have tenderness in this area even when the lumbosacral joint does not appear to be a significant part of the cause of the disability.

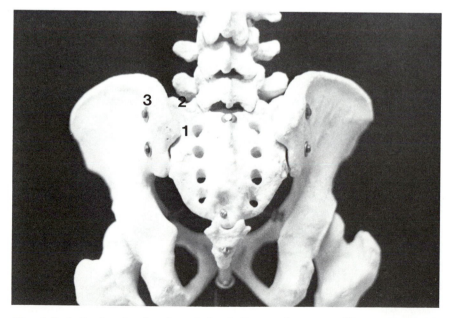

Fig. 4.8 Articulated pelvis from behind. (For explanation of figures see text.)

3. The third point is lateral to the PSIS (Fig. 4.8, 3). This can be associated with a gluteus medius trigger but is very common in those with back symptoms. It is not specifically associated with the sacroiliac joint and may sometimes be a sign of dysfunction even as high as the lower thoracic spine.

Chapter 5

Detailed Examination: The Spine

Spinal joints are examined to determine their mobility, the point in the normal range at which motion is restricted, and the presence or absence of abnormalities of tissue texture. The most important part of the tissue reaction is usually hypertonus in muscle. This, however, is not the only tissue affected and for this reason the term tissue texture abnormality (TTA) will be used in this edition.

Fully specific diagnosis depends on finding, for each abnormal joint, the precise position in its range of motion at which there is restriction. This must be established in all three planes, and it is worth noting at this point that the range, for instance, of left sidebending will be reduced if, when the movement is tested, the patient is more flexed than if the anteroposterior position had been nearer the neutral. Only when the location of the barrier is known will it be possible to position the patient at the barrier in all three planes in order to carry out specific treatment.

It follows from the above that, in almost any joint, the barrier is not a single point. The precise location will depend on whether flexion/extension, sidebending or rotation is introduced first and may also change depending on the amount of the initial movement that is introduced.

For many years of manipulative practice, one of the authors used what he now regards as a semispecific examination, and although he was then working with incomplete information, his results were by no means bad. The examination consisted of two basic parts, first testing for loss of mobility in an individual joint, and second, finding the location of the tight tissue. Perhaps it is worth pointing out again that, at first, the idea that it was possible to distinguish individual spinal joint mobility was a great surprise!

Some will find that the simpler approach is easier to start with and for this reason it has been retained in this edition. There is a close correlation between the findings of this and the fully specific approach but there are some patients in whom it is not good enough. It is recommended, therefore, that even if you start with the simpler approach, you should progress to the fully specific one as you gain experience.

To clear up any possible misunderstanding, flexion refers to forward tilting of the superior surface of the vertebra. Extension refers to backward tilting of the superior surface. Rotation is named by the side to which the anterior surface of the vertebra turns. Sidebending is named by the side to which the superior surface of the vertebra tilts. When a vertebra is said to be dysfunctional, this always refers to the joint between that vertebra and the one below.

SEMISPECIFIC DIAGNOSIS

In this method, the parameters examined are joint motion and tissue tension. The first sign that suggests the presence of joint dysfunction is loss of motion. If at the same segment there is an area of increased tension in soft tissue (primarily muscle), this is considered to be evidence of joint dysfunction for which manipulative treatment may be appropriate. It should hardly be necessary to remind the reader that there are other causes of back pain and for some of them manipulation, at least that using high velocity thrusting, might be dangerous. It is the responsibility of the manipulator to satisfy himself that such conditions are not present.

Lumbar spine

Examination for hypertonus

When one is trying to assess the presence of hypertonus in muscle it is important to have the side being examined uppermost. This means that it is necessary to repeat the examination on the other side and that it is not possible, in this position, to compare the two sides directly. There is an advantage in that the examination for motion loss is performed twice, once from each side. In difficult cases this may be useful. If it is necessary to compare the tissue tension directly on the two sides, the patient must be prone.

1. In order to examine the right side of the spine, the patient should lie on her left side. To help her relax, she should support her head on a pillow or on her flexed left arm.

2. You stand in front of her.

3. Ease her left shoulder forward a little. This will tilt her backwards slightly which makes it easier to control her movement.

4. Grasp her right leg and flex her knee and hip. The position of the leg can be controlled either by your left hand (Fig. 5.1) or by your abdomen (Fig. 5.2). The use of the abdomen allows you to monitor with both your index fingers, which is an advantage.

5. By moving your body sideways you can flex and extend her lumbar spine at the level under examination.

6. To assess muscle tension, monitor with one or two fingers over the lateral musculature. It is usually possible to feel through the longissimus and there may also be hypertonus in that muscle itself. Each level should be examined in turn. In the lumbar spine it is usually easier to feel the abnormality if you move your fingers gently from medial to lateral.

7. The examination is then repeated on the other side after turning the patient over.

This technique can be used to examine the lower thoracic spine up to about the ninth thoracic vertebra.

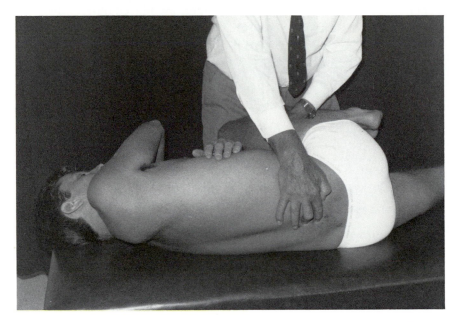

Fig. 5.1 Testing for motion in the lumbar spine using one hand to monitor.

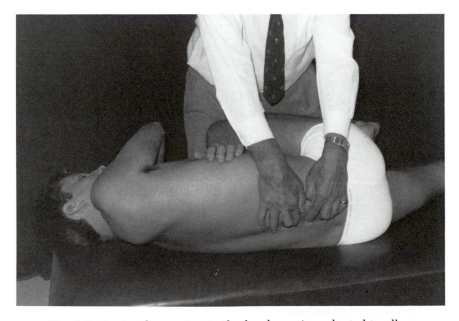

Fig. 5.2 Testing for motion in the lumbar spine adapted to allow use of both hands for monitoring.

Examination for loss of motion

1. The assessment of loss of motion uses the same position and movement of the patient but the examining fingers are placed differently.

2. Monitor with two (or more) fingers. One must be on the interspinous ligament of the joint in question, the other(s) should be on the interspinous interval of one or both of the neighbouring joints for comparison.

3. It need hardly be added that the amount of flexion of the patient's spine must be adjusted to bring the movement to the area being examined.

Thoracic spine

Examination for hypertonus

A variety of examination techniques is available, and necessary, for the assessment of muscle tension in the thoracic spine.

The lower few segments can be examined by the method described for the lumbar spine.

The mid-section is most easily examined prone, and the prone technique can also be used from the lower end up to about T3. When examining in this way, it is an advantage to have a hole or a slot in the table for the nose and chin because if the head is turned to one side it is much more difficult to compare one side with the other. This is more important when one tries to examine the higher joints. If the table is not so equipped, a cushion with a hole in it can be used.

The supine position can also be used. It has the disadvantage that only one side can be examined at one time but it is often easier for the patient to relax. The supine position is not so useful below about T8.

The sitting position is good for the upper section and can be used down to about T6. It is important to see that the patient does not 'slump' because if she does, she will restrict all motion. This sitting examination is a useful means of giving the patient some confidence, without which it will be difficult for her to relax. In the position to be described it is usually easy to find at least one level where there is hypertonus. This area will always be tender and, if a little extra pressure is applied, she will know both that there is something there and that you know how to find it. This is a great help to those who have been led to believe that they are making a fuss about nothing.

1. The prone examination.

(a) The patient lies prone with her head central, preferably with her nose and chin in a slot.

(b) You stand to either side and, using both hands, palpate the paraspinal muscles on each side at each level in turn. It is usually easier to assess abnormal tension in this region if one moves one's fingers up and down the spine rather than across the muscle fibres.

2. The supine examination (Fig. 5.3).

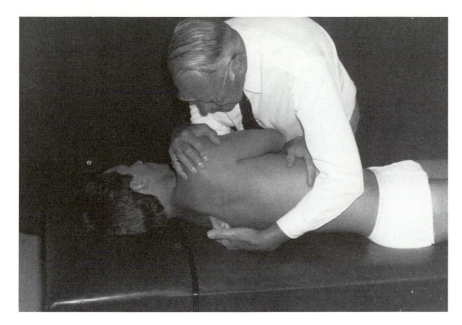

Fig. 5.3 Supine examination for hypertonus in the thoracic region.

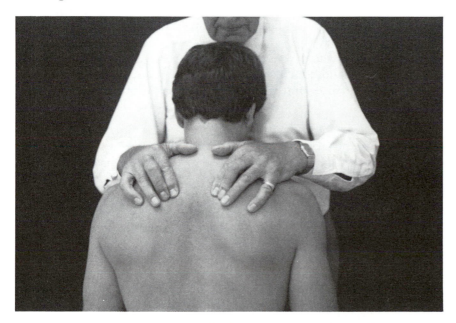

Fig. 5.4 Sitting examination for hypertonus in the upper thoracic region.

(a) The patient is supine with her head supported by a pillow.

(b) You stand to the side opposite to that which you wish to examine.

(c) To examine her left side you lift her left shoulder with your left hand and use your right hand to palpate the muscles at each level in turn.

(d) Repeat the examination from the other side.

3. The sitting examination (Fig. 5.4).

(a) The patient sits with her legs over the side of the table.

(b) Make sure that she is 'sitting up tall'.

(c) You stand in front, close enough for her to rest her forehead against the front of your chest.

(d) In this position you feel, with one or more fingers of each hand, for areas of hypertonus in the paraspinal muscles. Here also an up and down motion of the fingers is usually the most useful.

Examination for loss of motion

Motion testing may be done in flexion/extension, in sidebending or in rotation. When there is difficulty in interpreting the result of one test, it may be helpful to try one of the others.

The methods of testing will be described for the individual joint, but it is much easier to assess normality if one feels the motion at the next one or two levels as well. The screening examination will give you a good idea of the areas within which it is necessary to carry out this kind of detailed examination.

The different techniques to be described use the sitting position for the patient, except for one that is done prone. The main differences are in the grip adopted by the operator to control the patient and introduce the required motion. In all of them it is essential that the patient is relaxed. All techniques to be described are passive. You may monitor with either hand and use the other for inducing motion. For simplicity, the descriptions will assume that the left hand is the monitoring hand.

1. Sitting technique for flexion/extension from T3 to T12 (Fig. 5.5).

(a) You stand behind the patient who sits on a stool or with her legs over the side of the table.

(b) The patient laces her fingers together behind the base of her neck and allows her elbows to fall together in front. If she cannot do this, e.g. because of shoulder stiffness, see the next technique.

(c) Lift her elbows with your right hand and you will find that the amount that you lift them will determine the amount of flexion or extension of the thoracic spine.

(d) Monitor the supraspinous ligaments at each level in turn while you induce movement at those segments by lifting and lowering your right hand. At least two fingers should be used for monitoring so that the joint in question can be compared with its neighbours. At a normal segment it will be possible for you to feel the spinous processes open and close on flexion and extension respectively.

2. Variation for flexion/extension testing in a patient with a stiff shoulder (Fig. 5.6).

(a) The sitting position is the same.

(b) Assuming that she is unable to put her left hand on the back of her neck, the patient should put her right hand there and you thread your right forearm through her right axilla so that your hand rests on

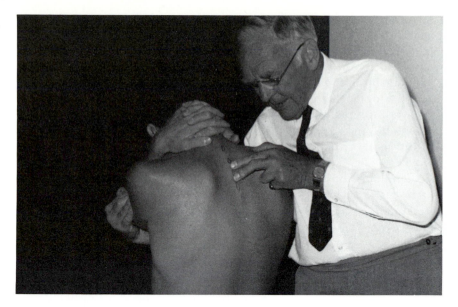

Fig. 5.5 Sitting examination for motion from T3 to T12.

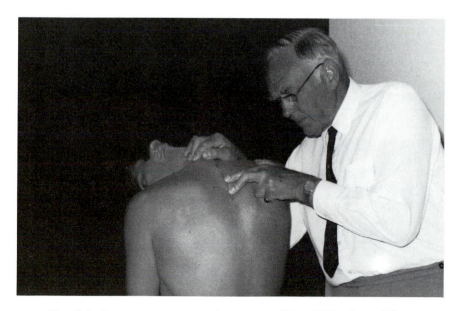

Fig. 5.6 Sitting examination for motion T3 to T12 adapted for a patient with a stiff shoulder.

top of her right hand on the back of her neck. If she can reach her right shoulder with her left hand, that will increase stability.

(c) Motion is introduced as before by movement of your right arm, and monitoring is as above.

(d) An alternative grip is for the patient to put her right hand on her left shoulder and for you to control motion by passing your left arm through her left axilla. You then grasp her right arm with your left hand.

3. Sitting technique for flexion/extension testing the upper thoracic spine, C7 to about T5 (Fig. 5.7).

(a) You stand behind the patient who sits on a stool or with her legs over the side of the table.

(b) Grasp the top of her head with your right hand so that you can induce flexion and extension by movement of the head and neck.

(c) Monitor, as above, with the fingers of your left hand on the supraspinous ligaments of two or more joints at one time.

4. Sitting technique for testing sidebending in the thoracic spine from T3 to T12.

(a) The position is the same as that for flexion/extension testing in the presence of a stiff shoulder except that the monitoring fingers are placed against the sides of the spinous processes, the better to feel the angulation of the upper on the lower at a mobile segment. Some will find it easier to use a thumb for monitoring for this movement.

(b) There are many variations. The alternative grip for the stiff shoulder examination above can be used. Another useful method is to place your right forearm on top of her right shoulder so that your hand lies across the back of her neck. Your index finger points towards her left shoulder and the remaining fingers curl around the base of her neck. Your thumb points down her back. This grip gives surprisingly good lateral control of movement (see Fig. 3.4, p. 45).

5. Sitting technique for testing rotation in the thoracic spine (Fig. 5.8). Either of the grips described for sidebending may be used. The monitoring fingers or thumb are placed at the side of the spinous processes to detect rotation between one and the next.

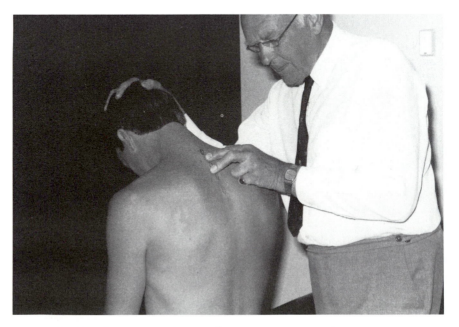

Fig. 5.7 Sitting examination for motion in upper thoracic spine.

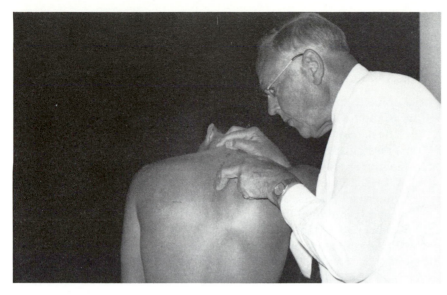

Fig. 5.8 Sitting examination for rotation in the thoracic spine.

6. Prone springing technique (Fig. 5.9).

(a) The patient lies prone.

(b) You stand beside her and the table should be low enough to allow your arms to be straight.

(c) With one or preferably both arms, you apply gentle springing pressure to each spinous process in turn. The pressure should be momentary and light, it is not desirable to produce an extension manipulation before making a diagnosis.

(d) If this springing causes pain and muscle spasm when performed gently, you should be alerted to the possibility that there is a destructive lesion at that level.

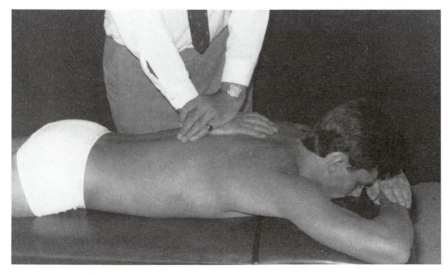

Fig. 5.9 Prone springing test for thoracic mobility.

Cervical spine

Examination for hypertonus

This may be done either with the patient sitting or with her supine.

1. Supine technique. This is better for the upper joints and is useful as low as about C6 (Fig. 5.10).
   (a) The patient lies supine with her head at the end of the table.
   (b) You stand at her head and support it with the palms of your hands or, often more easily, with your abdomen.
   (c) With the index and middle fingers of both hands you palpate for hypertonus at each level, on both sides at the same time.

2. Sitting technique. This can be used from C2 down and is better for joints below C6 (Fig. 5.11).
   (a) The patient sits on a stool or with her legs over the side of the table.
   (b) You stand in front, close enough for her to rest her head on your chest.
   (c) Use your index and middle fingers to feel the tension in the paraspinal muscles on both sides at each segment in turn. The tension abnormalities are more easily felt in the cervical region by a transverse movement of the finger pads across the muscle fibres. Sometimes a feeling of a ripple will be noticed at a segment with hypertonus, as if there were a bundle of tight cords.

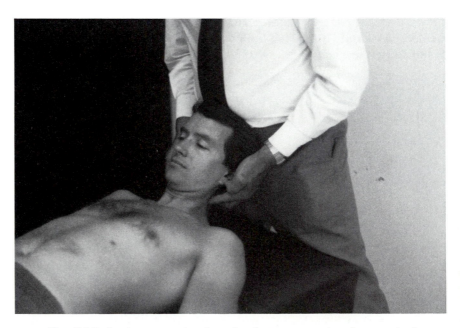

Fig. 5.10 Supine examination for hypertonus in the cervical region.

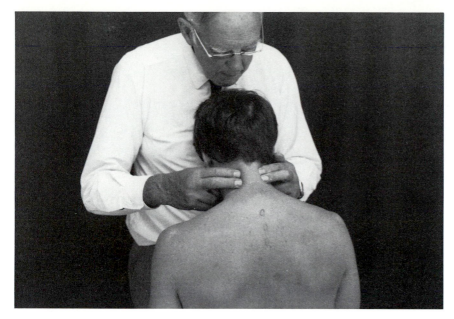

Fig. 5.11 Sitting examination for hypertonus in the cervical region.

Examination for loss of motion

The cervical spine is made up of two atypical and six typical joints, if C7–T1 is included.

Examination for sidebending restriction is the method recommended for the atypical occipitoatlantal and rotation restriction for the atlantoaxial joint. The very small size of the posterior tubercle of the atlas (it has no spinous process) makes the use of flexion/extension almost impossible. Sidebending can also be used in the remainder of the region but it becomes increasingly difficult below C6.

The technique used for estimating restriction of sidebending in any of these joints and the method of deducing the precise diagnosis from this information are described in the section on fully specific diagnosis in this region (see p. 88).

Estimation of flexion/extension restriction may be done in the typical joints (C2–T1) (Fig. 5.12).

1. The patient sits on a stool or with her legs over the side of the table.

2. You stand behind her and grasp her forehead with your right hand to control movement of the head and neck.

3. Monitor on two adjacent levels with thumb and index or index and middle fingers of your left hand over the interspinous intervals.

4. With your right hand, rock the head and neck in flexion and extension through the range that brings motion to the segment under examination.

5. Repeat at each joint.

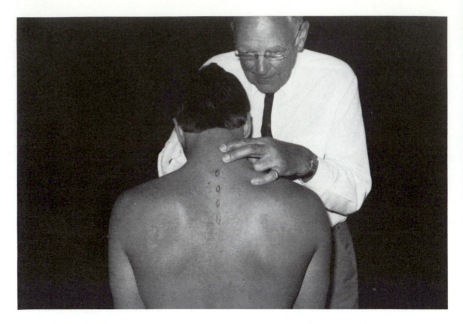

Fig. 5.12 Sitting examination for motion in the cervical region.

Estimation of sidebending and of rotation in the typical joints can be performed with the patient in the same position and a slight alteration of the position of the monitoring fingers.

POSITIONAL, FULLY SPECIFIC DIAGNOSIS

Before discussing techniques, it is important that certain characteristics of spinal motion are understood. In the lumbar and thoracic regions of the spine two different types of dysfunction occur. The common symptom-producing one is what has been called type II and is usually traumatic in origin. The restriction is of either flexion or extension with sidebending and rotation to the same side. The other is type I and is always found as a group of three or more. This dysfunction is often compensatory and may resolve when the primary cause has been treated. Type I occurs in neutral so that sidebending and rotation are to opposite sides.

In the cervical spine the situation is more complex. In the typical cervical joints, sidebending and rotation are always to the same side. This is the result of the facing of the facets and the fact that they are always in close apposition. At the atlantoaxial joint there is little movement other than rotation and the motion cannot be described as either type I or type II. At the occipitoatlantal joint the main movement is flexion/extension but there is a small range of sidebending which is always associated with a very small range of rotation to the opposite side (type I).

Facet and transverse process motion

This must be understood in order to interpret the findings of the types of positional examination which will be described. When the superior vertebra flexes on the one below, the inferior facets of the upper vertebra slide upwards and the vertebra translates forwards through a small distance which will vary with the obliquity of the facets at that level. As this happens the transverse processes also slide upwards and forwards. This motion can be felt if the fingers are in the right place and are not pressing too firmly. As the transverse process slides forward it becomes less easy to feel.

When the movement is sidebending to the left, the right facet of the superior vertebra will slide up and the right transverse process will ride up and become less prominent. Because the left facet joint remains closed, the left transverse process remains low and prominent posteriorly.

By following the movement of the transverse processes or, in the neck, of the lateral masses of the vertebrae, it is possible to determine precisely where there is a barrier to movement at any particular joint. The transverse processes of the cervical vertebrae are small, rather far anterior and usually very tender; for this reason the part of the bone used is the lateral mass or articular pillar. In some patients it is possible to feel the actual facets in the thoracic spine. The differential movement of the facets gives the same information as that of the transverse processes.

It is also possible to deduce the position of the barrier by a static method. This is done by noting the relative positions of the transverse processes in neutral, flexion and extension.

To define the restriction of motion

Thoracic and lumbar

1. Static.
(a) Observation is made of the rotation of the transverse processes at the segment in question. This is done with the patient in neutral. She is then flexed in the knee–elbow position or as in the sitting forward flexion test and the rotation is again noted. Finally she is extended in the sphinx position and the rotation noted once more. The observations may be made in any order.
(b) If in neutral, the transverse processes are level or the left one is more posterior, and this rotation is exaggerated in extension but levelled in flexion; it means that the right facet will not close and that there is a barrier to extension and rotation to the right.
(c) If in neutral, the transverse processes are level or rotated left (the left one is more posterior), and this rotation is exaggerated by flexion but levelled in extension; it means that the left facet will not open and that there is a barrier to flexion and rotation to the right. In the diagrams in Fig. 5.13, the differences have been exaggerated for clarity. The clinical

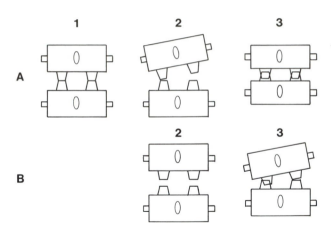

Fig. 5.13 Diagram to show movement of facets. In column 1 the spine is in neutral. In column 2 the spine is forward flexed. In column 3 the spine is extended. In line A there is restriction of flexion at the left facet joint. This automatically causes left sidebending (and left rotation) of the upper vertebra on the lower. In extension, both facet joints close fully. In line B there is normal opening on flexion but the right facet joint fails to close. This also produces left sidebending and left rotation of the upper vertebra on the lower.

feel of the situation depicted in A2 is the same as that in B3. The differentiation depends on what the rotation is in the other positions.

(d) If in neutral, the transverse processes are rotated left and they remain unlevel in either flexion or extension; it means that there is either a neutral (type I) dysfunction or an anatomical asymmetry. The difference can be determined by two further observations. First, if there is a neutral lesion, there will be a group of at least three vertebrae rotated in the same sense. Second, if there is an anatomical asymmetry, there will be no change in the amount of rotation on changing position, whereas with a neutral lesion the amount of rotation will vary as the position is changed.

(e) Asymmetry which does not change on flexion and extension can also be due to bilateral problems at the same joint. It happens when the joint on one side is stuck with the facets open and the joint on the other side is stuck with the facets closed. The differential diagnosis is made by testing for movement between the spinous processes. The anatomically asymmetrical joint will have normal motion. The abnormal will not move.

2. Dynamic (Fig. 5.14).

(a) Observation is made of the difference in the movement of the transverse processes on the two sides when the segment under examination is moved from neutral to flexion and to extension. In the lower cervical spine the articular pillars are used instead. Active movement

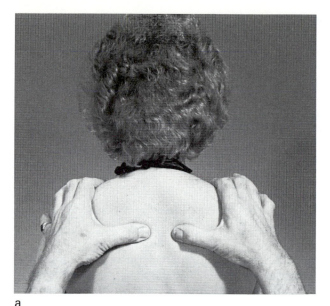

a

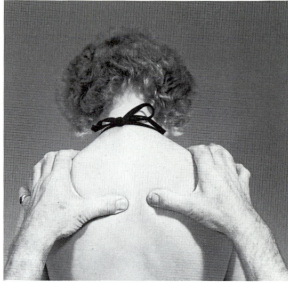

b

Fig. 5.14 Dynamic position testing in the thoracic spine. **(a)** Thumbs placed on transverse processes of T3 in neutral flexion. **(b)** In forward flexion of this area the right thumb rides up but the left remains down and more prominent (indicating failure of the left facet joint to open). **(c)** In extension the thumbs ride down and back equally.

c

is preferable as this allows examination with both hands. If passive movement is used, the transverse processes must be contacted by the index and middle fingers of the free hand, which is less easy than the use of both index fingers or both thumbs. Increased prominence of one transverse process indicates a failure of flexion on that side and can also be used in diagnosis.

(b) The patient sits on a stool or on the side of the table with her feet supported.

(c) The index fingers or thumbs are used to find the groove lateral to the longissimus muscle on each side, between it and the iliocostalis. It is important to use pressure that is as light as possible in this examination, although it must be enough to locate the bony points. The corresponding rib is found and the finger or thumb is moved a short distance medially to find the tip of the transverse process.

(d) The patient is asked to bend forwards. For the upper thoracic joints it is enough to ask her to look down at her feet. In the lower lumbar region almost full flexion may be needed. The observation is easier if the movement is not too fast.

(e) The patient is then asked to look up at the ceiling and, for lower joints, to arch her back as well.

(f) The argument is as follows.

(i) If on forward flexion the left transverse process is level with that on the right but on extension it fails to descend and becomes less prominent, it indicates a failure of the left facet joint to close fully. The corresponding barrier is to extension and to sidebending and rotation to the left.

(ii) If on forward flexion the left transverse process is lower and more prominent than the right (i.e. the right transverse process has risen vertically and moved forward more than the left) and on extension the transverse processes become level and equally prominent, it indicates a failure of the left facet joint to open fully. The corresponding barrier is to flexion and to sidebending and rotation to the right.

(iii) With a neutral dysfunction there will be some irregularity of motion and the transverse processes will not become even in any position.

3. Sidebending has been omitted from this discussion because it is coupled to rotation (one way or the other) and it is the rotation which is more easily felt.

Cervical

The occipitoatlantal and atlantoaxial joints are atypical. They move together and each has its own characteristics. At the upper joint there is a wide range of flexion and extension and a small range of sidebending associated with a very small range of rotation.[1] At the lower joint there is a wide range of rotation, a small range of flexion and extension but almost no sidebending.

1. The dynamic method described above may be used with advantage for the lower two or three cervical joints.

2. For the remaining typical joints, sidebending is the easiest method (Fig. 5.15).

(a) The patient lies supine.

(b) You stand or sit at her head and palpate the lateral masses (articular pillars) of the cervical vertebrae with the tips of your fingers. At the same time you use the palms of your hands to lift her head. The lateral masses are found laterally, in front of the posterior muscle group.

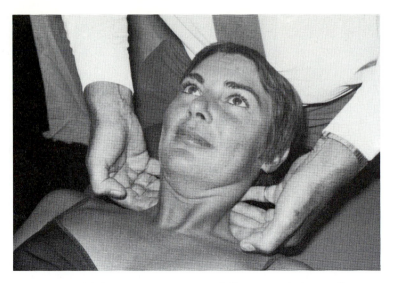

Fig. 5.15 Examination to define restriction of motion in the cervical spine, C2 to C7.

The transverse processes are a little further in front and are very tender.

(c) By a translatory motion introduced by your fingertips, sidebend each level in turn both to left and to right. This should be done both in flexion and extension. If in flexion C4 will not translate to the right, but moves freely to the left, and at the same time in extension it moves both ways, it means that there is restriction of left sidebending (and therefore of left rotation) and restriction of flexion of C4 on C5. In other words, the *right* facet will not open.

(d) If the restriction had been worse in extension but free in flexion, it would mean that the *left* facet would not close. There would have been a barrier to extension and left sidebending (and rotation).

(e) If one places the fingers correctly, one can feel four different vertebrae at the same time. This is useful both because it allows one to determine the level very quickly and because one can scan rapidly to find which level has a restriction. The small finger should be placed just below the 2nd cervical vertebra, on the lateral mass of the 3rd. The other fingers will then fall naturally onto the 4th, 5th and 6th vertebrae. When using this method it is wise to attempt translation at one level at a time by moving only one pair of fingers.

(f) The localisation of the level of the restriction can also be done from below. To do this you first identify the 7th cervical spinous process and then place your index fingers on the lateral mass of the 6th, which will allow your remaining fingers to find the 5th, 4th and 3rd vertebrae.

3. For the atlantoaxial joint, rotation is used (Fig. 5.16).

(a) The patient lies supine.

(b) You stand or sit at her head.

(c) With both your hands, lift her head into almost full neck flexion. Do not fully flex the head on the neck. This position very much reduces

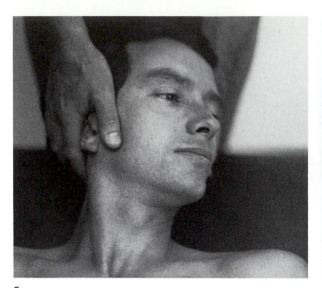 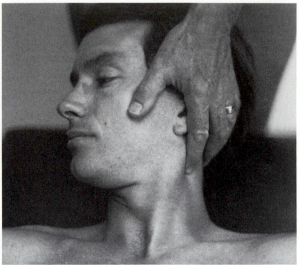

a   b

Fig. 5.16 (a) and **(b)** Examination for restriction of motion in the C1–2 joint.

the component of neck rotation which occurs in the typical joints. In neutral flexion/extension this may be half the total rotation.

(d) Rotate her head gently to the barrier in each direction. Normally the movement is symmetrical and may be as much as 75°. Note any asymmetry.

4. For the occipitoatlantal joint, the movement tested is sidebending (Fig. 5.17).

(a) The patient lies supine.

(b) You stand or sit at her head.

(c) Lift her head with one of your hands on either side. Tilt the chin down to produce flexion at the joint. Do not force this movement.

(d) Translate her head first to one side then to the other and observe how far the midline of the head moves away from the midline of the trunk (the nose is a convenient marker) (Fig. 5.17a and b). It helps to find the end-point if one monitors on the sides of the C1–2 joint with the index fingers. In a normal joint the movement is usually more than 13 mm (0.5 inch). It should be symmetrical. Note that the movement which you introduce is translation *not* sidebending.

(e) Repeat the test with the occipitoatlantal joint in slight extension, produced by tipping the head gently upwards. Excessive extension must be avoided (Fig. 5.17c and d).

(f) A false positive test is not uncommon. In order to produce translation, not only must the joint itself be able to sidebend but the lower neck joints must also be able to bend to the opposite side. If this is suspected, the test should be repeated after the lower joints have been treated.

5. For those unfamiliar with this use of the term, translation in this context signifies a side to side movement without tilting of the long axis of the part. Note that if translation to the left is restricted, it signifies

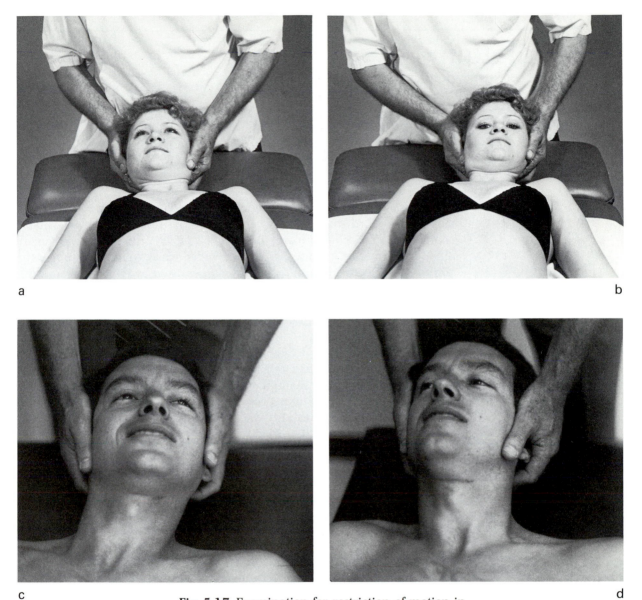

Fig. 5.17 Examination for restriction of motion in
the occipitoatlantal joint: **(a)** and **(b)** in flexion, **(c)**
and **(d)** in extension.

a loss of right sidebending at the occipitoatlantal joint in either flexion
or extension. The latter depends on the sagittal plane position in which
the side to side motion was tested.

REFERENCE

1. Kapandji I. A. (1974). *The Physiology of the Joints*, Vol. 3, 2nd edn. Edinburgh: Churchill Livingstone.

Chapter 6

Manipulation

Nomenclature and terminology

There is at the present time disagreement as to the breadth of the meaning of the word manipulation. In Europe the term is reserved almost entirely for procedures involving a high velocity, thrusting movement. In North America it is used in a much wider sense, to include any active or passive movement initiated, assisted or resisted by the physician. This includes treatment sometimes listed as articulation or mobilisation, isometric and isotonic contraction techniques and even the so-called functional or indirect techniques where no force at all is applied by the physician.

In the *Shorter Oxford English Dictionary* (2nd edn, 1939) manipulation is defined in part as: '(3) The handling of objects for a particular purpose; in surgery the manual examination of a part of the body. Also, manual action.' There does not appear to be any justification, in the English language at least, for the narrow interpretation of the word, and in this volume it will be used in the wide or North American sense.

The term **muscle energy** is used here to cover the techniques which were described in the third edition, mostly under the term isometric. Many of these techniques are isometric but some are isotonic or a combination of the two, and as the basic principles are similar it is better to bring them together under one term.

The notation used to describe the precise position of the joint needs to be explained. The capitals FRS or ERS are used to signify the position in which the joint is found: E and F stand for extension and flexion, respectively; R stands for rotation and S for sidebending. The R and S are followed by a subscript denoting the side to which the joint is held. The old convention used R and S separately because the same type of notation was used for neutral lesions where the rotation and sidebend are to opposite sides. The more modern convention is used in this book: neutral lesions are described by N followed by a subscript which denotes the side of the convexity of the curve. In the descriptions of techniques that follow, both the notation and the written description of the position are given.

TYPES OF MANIPULATION

Many different techniques have been used to alter or remove the restrictive barrier and its associated abnormal tissue tension. In the early editions of this book only high velocity thrusting techniques were described, and some of them were quite non-specific. The latter were omitted altogether from the third edition as being inadequate.

Specific high velocity techniques are the great standby and have been in use for more than a hundred years. Unfortunately, however, they are not without disadvantage and, occasionally hazard. In recent years a significant number of vascular accidents have occurred during high velocity treatment of the upper neck and this form of treatment is better avoided. If for any reason it is decided that thrusting treatment of the upper neck is essential, it would be wise to make sure that the patient understands that there can be a significant risk.

Techniques which do not involve the application of anything other than resistive external force have advantages. This is especially true in the aged, in the osteoporotic, in those in whom the pain is too severe to permit a thrusting procedure and in those who are sick (if for any reason it is thought advisable to treat an area of somatic dysfunction at that time).

All these techniques require that the joint be examined and treated as an entity, separate from its neighbours. The concept that it is possible to do this is foreign to those brought up in most orthodox medical schools. Furthermore, if it is accepted that it might be possible, it is thought that only a special few can learn the necessary skills. Bearing in mind James Mennell's warning (quoted in Chapter 1), these techniques are such that they can be learned by anyone who is prepared to find the time and make the effort.

High velocity, low amplitude manipulation

In this method the location of the restrictive barrier is found and, by a combination of positioning and application of external force, the joint is moved through the barrier, if possible all the way to the end of its normal range of motion. Obviously the force must be controlled so that it does not push the joint beyond the anatomical barrier or damage will result. This is one of the difficulties. The amount of movement required is small and occasionally the force needed may be considerable. The better one's localisation, or the more accurately the barrier is engaged, the less the force that is required.

The lever principle can be used with advantage. If it is possible to apply the force through a long lever, the strength of the force is divided and the distance travelled is multiplied by the ratio of the length of the long lever to that of the shorter one. This has the double benefit of reducing the force needed and increasing the distance moved at the point where it is applied. The application of the principle will be illustrated in descriptions of actual high velocity techniques.

Mobilisation or articulation

In this method the barrier is once again found but this time, instead of forcing the joint through it, the barrier is almost caressed. By taking the joint gently up to the barrier, moving along or beside it (if such motion is available) and then away again, the barrier is encouraged to recede. It will often do so and, if motion is gained, the process can be repeated several times.

Actual techniques for doing this will not be described here, but those interested can find them in several sources.[1,2,3]

Muscle energy techniques

These were described in the third edition under the heading of isometrics. In this edition the muscle energy term is used because many of the techniques are not strictly or not solely isometric.

Muscle energy techniques are direct techniques. Like those employing high velocity, they work with the joint taken up to the barrier. The chief difference is that instead of the barrier being forced to let go by a thrust applied by the operator, the patient's own muscles are made to work in a way that causes the barrier to recede.

One of the problems with muscle energy techniques is that the barrier must be found and accurately engaged in all three planes before they are likely to succeed. This makes accuracy of diagnosis and in positioning very important. This degree of accuracy is not easy for those beginning to do this kind of work.

The reason for the success of muscle energy techniques is probably that in some way the resisted muscle effort resets the 'gain' in the gamma system which controls the moment-by-moment length of the muscle fibres. The spindle is 'cheated' into thinking that the muscle has shortened during the contraction and, on relaxation, allows some lengthening. In isometric contractions it is most important that the counterforce should be equal to the force exerted by the patient and, therefore, unyielding. Failure to maintain the position, and failure to reach the barrier accurately, will make the treatment less effective.

Maximal contraction of the muscles is not required for this method of joint treatment. It is very often necessary to caution the patient not to use too much force. The tightness is usually in muscles that are quite small. If much force is used, accessory muscles will be brought in and this will detract from the effectiveness of the treatment on the specific tissues that need to be made to relax.

There are other uses for muscle energy techniques. They can be used, for example, to stretch peripheral muscle such as the hamstrings or to strengthen weak muscles and increase the tone in those that have been stretched. They are also effective in overcoming joint contracture after immobilisation. For some of these applications much stronger contractions may be called for. If the anatomy of any muscle is known, it is possible to devise a muscle energy procedure to stretch it.

Other types of manipulation

There are a number of other ways in which dysfunctional joints can be treated. Maigne[3] uses a type of exaggeration movement. The joint is positioned away from the barrier and the thrust is in the direction of ease. The treatment is successful in many cases, although the reason for its success is not known with certainty.

There are also what are known as indirect techniques. In the best known of these the joint is taken to the point of maximum ease, that is to say, the point at which the tension in the tissues around the joint is at a minimum, and is held there. After a short time (30–90 seconds), the tissue tensions begin to change. When the changes begin it is most important that they should be followed by the operator so that the joint is kept as closely as possible at its point of maximum ease. In a relatively short time the tensions may relax altogether and the treatment is over.

The indirect treatments are of particular value in those who are seriously ill and in those where the condition is so acute that no other treatment is possible.

LOCALISATION OF FORCE

A cabinet maker does not drive home a nail all the way with a simple hammer, if he did he would mark the wood around the hole with the final blows. He uses a nail punch to finish the job so that there is only a small hole to fill instead of the mark of the face of the hammer.

In the same way a manipulator localises the force to the joint that is to be moved, otherwise neighbouring structures might be harmed. One of the reasons for the scant success of traction is that it cannot be accurately localised. It wastes most, and often all, of its effect on neighbouring mobile joints and may have little or no effect on the one causing the trouble. Marked separation can often be seen at normal joints if x-rays are taken while the patient is on traction.

The force is localised by positioning the patient. The third law tells us that movement of the spine away from neutral in any plane will limit the range of motion in the other planes. This can be applied in such a way that on either side of the lesion, movement of the joints is prevented in the direction of the intended force. This procedure is known as locking and the concept involved is helpful when one is considering high velocity manipulation. The concept of locking is not the same as that of the barrier described in Chapter 3. Locking is what one can do to a normal joint. The restrictive barrier is what one finds in an abnormal joint. It is clear, however, that locking involves taking the normal joint up to one part of its physiological, or even to the anatomical, barrier.

Locking can be produced by taking movement in any plane as far as it will go, e.g. flexion. It can also be produced by movement in a combination of planes. The division of body movement into three planes at right angles to each other is a descriptive device which nature does not recognise. Locking will occur in any combination of rotation and sidebending with or without flexion or extension, provided that the movement is taken to its limit in that direction.

Here, however, is a difficulty. Spinal joints do not move separately, they are like traffic lights that are linked together. Long before the first joint reaches the limit of its movement, the next one has started to move. It is easy to go too far and at least partially lock the joint that one is trying to move. One of the things that one learns by experience is how far to go. In order to decide how far to go one must monitor with one's fingers. Monitoring can be by either or both of two changes: first, the movement of the joint, second, the tissue tension around the joint. Accuracy in this kind of palpation is much improved by practice.

All movements must be made by the manipulator with the patient relaxed. Any attempt to help on the part of the patient will make it impossible for the manipulator to feel accurately.

For a start the following method is useful. When positioning the patient by whatever method is appropriate, the movement is continued until the tissue tension at the problem joint is felt to increase. Alternatively, one might say until the problem joint ought to move as judged by the movement of the joint above and that below. At that point one reverses the movement slightly so that the tissue tension at the *next* level begins to relax or the movement at the *next* level is partly undone. By 'the next level' is meant the next joint in the direction from which locking is being produced, e.g. if one is locking up to L2–3 from below (in order to manipulate the L2–3 joint), the tension and movement should be partly taken out from the L3–4 joint. The commonest mistake among beginners is to go too far and make their task more difficult by locking the problem joint.

APPLICATION OF FORCE

Nature has equipped the vertebrae with a number of small levers by which they can be moved. The most useful are the transverse and spinous processes in the lumbar and thoracic regions and the articular pillars (articular or lateral masses) in the neck.

The total range of movement at a single spinal joint is variable but always small (see Chapter 2 for figures). Some force may be required in order to overcome the stiffness and make the joint move. In order to avoid damage, the force must be stopped as soon as the movement has occurred. This is difficult with a short lever but, if one can use a longer lever, not only is the strength of the force reduced but also the distance travelled is increased, making the procedure doubly easier. Such a lever can be constructed by accurate locking of the joints above and/or below the lesion.

Flexion or extension can be used to lock the joints and one or other is the usual method in the lumbar spine. It does make a difference if one uses the most appropriate. If there is restriction of flexion, it is better to lock up to the lesion by flexion, with or without other plane movements. This is because in such a dysfunction, correction of the sagittal plane part of the restriction is important. Clearly, if one applies a force to a joint to move it when the next joint both above and below is in flexion, the problem joint will tend to flex. This is appropriate for a flexion restriction but not if the loss is of extension, in that case the sagittal plane component of the locking position should be extension. It is often better to use a somewhat different position for locking from above down to that used from below up. If, for instance, simple flexion is used both above and below, a small movement of the patient might easily result in the problem joint being itself brought into flexion locking.

There are techniques for applying high velocity, low amplitude thrust directly to the transverse or spinous processes (or to the articular pillars in the neck). These are short lever techniques. When using such a technique, it is important that the amplitude of (distance travelled by) the force should be very strictly controlled. Long lever techniques, when available, are often easier on both operator and patient. Hybrid techniques will also be described in which the lever on one side is long and that on the other is short. These can be very useful and if possible the force should be applied to the long lever side.

SUBSEQUENT VISITS

A successful manipulation will alter the patient's condition and it may well be that different manipulations will be required. It is essential that a thorough examination is made on each visit before any treatment is given.

It is not pleasant to talk of one's mistakes, but in some patients the signs are difficult to interpret and it is possible for even an experienced manipulator to find, on a subsequent visit, that the joint previously treated was, for instance, that next to the one that now needs treatment, and that probably one's previous assessment had been incorrect. A single treatment at the 'wrong' level may well result in symptomatic improvement, but if it is done several times it usually makes the symptoms worse again.

A patient whose condition, when first seen, is very acute will have widespread muscle spasm, making localised diagnosis difficult.

Those, like so many, who have had previous trouble may respond well initially to treatment of a new problem. Often, however, it will be necessary to find and treat the remaining dysfunctions from the old problems before the new one will remain better.

RE-EXAMINATION

It is always good practice to re-examine the joint after doing a manipulation. It is only by re-examination that one can find out if the object of the manipulation has been achieved. This is particularly true of muscle energy treatment where the 'cavitation' sound is the exception rather than the rule. If there is no change, some other procedure or a repeat treatment may be helpful.

REFERENCES

1. Stoddard A. (1959). *Manual of Osteopathic Technique*. London: Hutchinson.
2. Maitland G. D. (1964). *Vertebral Manipulation*. London: Butterworth.
3. Maigne R. (1972). *Orthopaedic Medicine*. Springfield, Ill: Charles C Thomas.

Chapter 7

Treatment of the Joints of the Pelvis

PRIORITIES

The authors have changed slightly the recommended order of treatment. The present suggested order of treatment in the low back is as follows.

Fully specific approach

1. Pubic malalignment.
(a) Superior pubis.
(b) Inferior pubis.
(c) Separated pubis.
2. Superior innominate shear, or the rare inferior shear.
3. Sacroiliac dysfunctions. *But if there is a maladapted lumbar lesion, this should be treated first.*
(a) Anterior torsion.
(b) Posterior torsion.
(c) Inferior sacral shear.
(d) Superior sacral shear.
4. Lumbar dysfunctions, including the lowest thoracic joints.
(a) Type II lesions.
(b) Any remaining type I lesions.
5. Iliosacral dysfunctions (except the innominate shears which should have been dealt with before).
(a) Posterior innominate.
(b) Anterior innominate.
(c) Inflare and outflare.
6. Note that pelvic dysfunctions are commonly multiple and that posterior torsion is almost always associated with other pelvic problems that will need treatment. This is one good reason for getting into the habit of testing again after treatment to see if something more is required. The forward flexion tests should be done again every time after a pubic dysfunction or iliac shear has been corrected.

Simplified approach

Although one of the authors was originally taught to treat the pelvis first, a greater understanding of the effect of muscles on the pelvis does suggest that it is better to treat the lumbar spine before treating the pelvis by this method. If the function of the lumbar region can be restored to near normal by treating the intervertebral joints, it will sometimes be found that the pelvic problem has resolved. The exception is pubic asymmetry, which should always come first.

An additional reason for treating the lumbar spine first is that occasionally severe distress can be precipitated if the pelvis is treated first when there are acute problems in the lumbar spine.

Many of the pelvic dysfunctions that we see will respond to the simplified approach but there will be some that require the fully specific treatment. It is probable that a number of those who do respond would have done so more quickly if the specific approach had been used.

CLINICAL METHODS

Simplified approach

In the pelvis some of the same tests are used and the more that is found out, the more likely it is that the treatment will be successful.

1. The forward flexion tests are used as the primary indication of pelvic dysfunction. Other sacroiliac motion tests may also be used if necessary.

2. The diagnosis of pubic dysfunction depends on the finding of asymmetry. Occasionally a pubic asymmetry will be found with negative forward flexion tests (FFTs). In that case the side can be determined by the presence of tenderness and TTA at the pubic tubercle, at the insertion of the inguinal ligament. If there is doubt about the TTA, the direct motion test may be done.

3. After the pubis has been treated, the lumbar and lowest thoracic joints are next examined and dysfunctions dealt with (see Chapter 8).

4. The pelvis is then re-examined starting with the FFTs and, if asymmetrical, it is treated by correcting the innominate rotation.

5. In all cases it is wise to check the gluteal region for hypertonic muscle and to treat tightness, especially in the pyriformis and gluteus medius and minimus. Other thigh muscles may also need to be balanced.

Fully specific approach

Diagnosis has been dealt with in Chapter 5, and the differentiating points only will be mentioned with each separate condition in this chapter.

Although the remaining iliosacral dysfunctions come at the end of the priorities, the innominate shears will be dealt with early because their treatment should take precedence over anything else except pubic dysfunctions. Each treatment will be described for one side only. For the other side it is only necessary to reverse the labels.

Pubis

1. Superior pubis on the left, diagnosis.
(a) Standing FFT, usually positive left.
(b) Left pubis does not move well.
(c) Pubic tubercle (and superior ramus) high left.
(d) Inguinal ligament, tender and TTA at insertion.
Superior pubis on the left, treatment (Fig. 7.1).
(a) The patient is supine with her left buttock at the edge of the table so that her PSIS is still just on the table.
(b) You stand on her left, facing her head, and hold her left leg just above the ankle between your legs. Alternatively you stand on one leg and support her ankle by bending your other knee so that her ankle rests on yours.
(c) Lean forward enough to rest your left hand on her right ASIS to stabilise her position on the table.
(d) With your right hand on her lower thigh, press her left leg down gently as far as it easily goes (to the barrier).
(e) The patient should attempt to raise her left leg while you prevent movement with your right hand.
(f) After 4 or 5 seconds you both relax, but you maintain the position. Note that most patients only stop pushing at the first request and a further instruction is needed before they relax fully. Full relaxation is essential for successful muscle energy treatment.
(g) When she has relaxed fully, you gently 'take up the slack' by pressing down on her leg while you allow her ankle to drop as far as is appropriate.
(h) When you have reached the new barrier, repeat steps (e), (f) and (g) two or three times and then re-examine the pubic position.

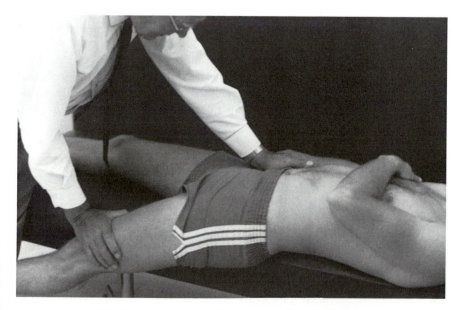

Fig. 7.1 Treatment of superior pubis on the left.

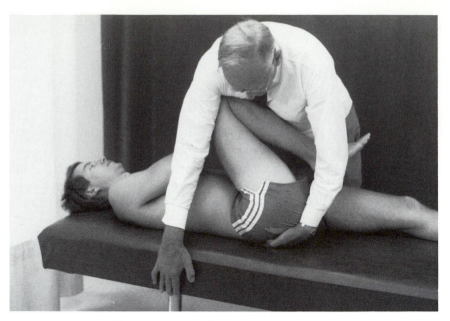

Fig. 7.2 Treatment of inferior pubis on the right.

2. Inferior pubis on the right, diagnosis.
(a) Standing FFT, usually positive right.
(b) Right pubis does not move well.
(c) Pubic tubercle, low right.
(d) Inguinal ligament, tender and TTA at insertion.
Inferior pubis on the right, treatment (Fig. 7.2).
(a) The patient is supine with her right hip and knee fully flexed. You need to be able to resist the movement of her leg with your trunk. The usual method is to lean over her and put her right knee in your right axilla.

(b) You stand on her left and slide your left hand under her buttock so that your index finger reaches the lateral side of her right PSIS and your middle finger is in the sulcus between the sacrum and ilium. You can then monitor to see that you do not flex her leg too far and 'bind' the sacroiliac joint.

(c) With the palm of your left hand, you pull on her ischial tuberosity in the direction of the pubic symphysis.

(d) With your right hand, you either press down on her right ASIS or grip the table to stabilise your position.

(e) The patient should attempt to push her right foot towards the foot of the table, or simply 'try to push me away'. The force must be controlled or you will not be able to prevent movement.

(f) Both relax, but you maintain the position. (See note on relaxation under treatment of superior pubis.)

(g) When she has fully relaxed, you take up the slack by increasing the hip flexion. Monitor with your left hand and stop before the sacrum begins to move.

(h) When you have reached the new barrier, repeat steps (e), (f) and (g) two or three times and then re-examine.

3. Blunderbuss treatment for pubic dysfunction (Fig. 7.3). This can be used for superior or inferior subluxations. Its success depends on the tendency of the bones to return to their normal position if the tight muscle is made to relax. The second part is appropriate for separations at the symphysis.

(a) The patient is supine with both knees bent up so that her feet are on the table close to her buttocks.

(b) You stand to either side and place one of your forearms so that you hold her knees apart between your dorsiflexed hand and your elbow. (Holding them apart by your two hands is unnecessarily hard work!) The patient should attempt to bring her knees together firmly. This can be repeated if necessary.

(c) Next, she should bring her knees together and you hold them there by locking both your arms round them. She should try to separate her knees against your resistance. This also may be repeated (Fig. 7.3b).

Innominate shears

1. Superior innominate shear on the left, diagnosis.

(a) Standing FFT, positive left. If in doubt, confirm by one of the other tests for sacroiliac mobility. When it is possible to determine this, it will be found that both the superior and the inferior poles of the sacroiliac joint are immobile.

(b) Iliac crest, left high, both supine and prone.

(c) Ischial tuberosity, left high by more that 7 mm (0.25 inch).

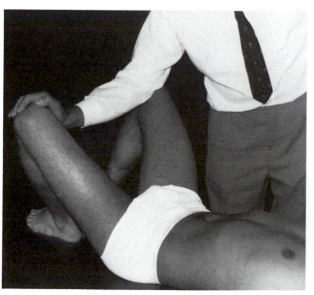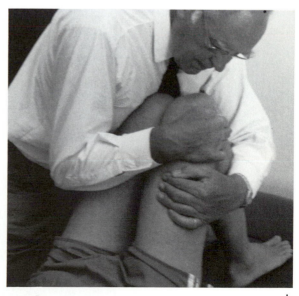

a
b

Fig. 7.3 Blunderbuss treatment of pubic dysfunction: **(a)** to separate, **(b)** to approximate.

(d) Sacrotuberous ligament, slack on the left.

(e) Medial malleoli, left short both prone and supine.

Superior innominate shear on the left, treatment (Fig. 7.4).

(a) The patient is supine.

(b) You stand at her feet and block her right leg from movement towards you.

(c) Pick up her left leg, holding above the ankle, and find the position in adduction–abduction that appears to 'loose-pack' the sacroiliac joint. This is in order to make the joint move more easily. At the same time, internally rotate enough to 'close-pack' (and thus protect) the hip joint.

(d) Pull steadily on her left leg while she does forced breathing in and out. This will help to rock loose the sacrum.

(e) At the end of the third exhalation, she should give a cough, and as she does this, you give a sharp tug on her left leg.

(f) Re-examine.

(g) Sometimes the superior innominate shear will tend to recur on weightbearing. If recurrence occurs, first check the pubic bones for position once again. If these are normal, it is best for the patient to wear a cinch-type sacroiliac belt. This should be worn whenever she is out of bed for the first six weeks and thereafter until the reduction is maintained at the next visit. The belt should be about 5 cm (2 inches) wide and must be worn below the iliac crests and above the symphysis.

2. Inferior innominate shear on the right (rare), diagnosis.

(a) Standing FFT, positive right.

(b) *All other parameters are the same as if there were a superior innominate shear on the left.*

(c) If necessary, confirm the side (and therefore the direction) by one

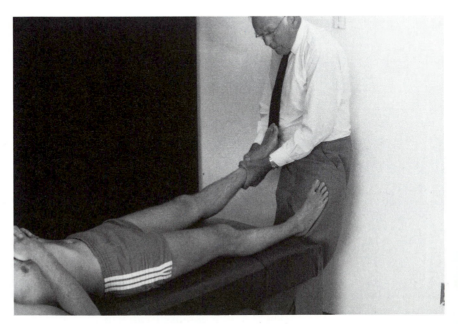

Fig. 7.4 Treatment of superior innominate shear.

of the other tests for sacroiliac stiffness. In this case, also both poles of the joint will be immobile.

Inferior innominate shear on the right, treatment (Fig. 7.5a and b).

(a) The patient lies on her left side.

(b) You stand behind her and lift her right leg. Place your right hand so that your thumb is medial to her right ischial tuberosity and your index finger is in contact with her right pubic rami. Your forearm should support her thigh.

(c) Place your left hand so that your thumb is medial to the posterior

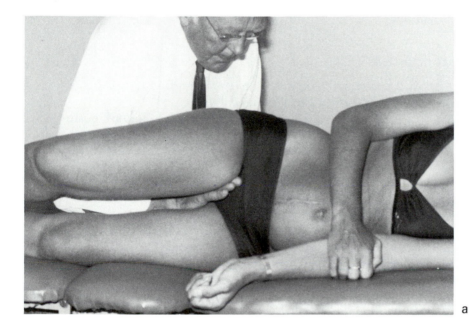

a

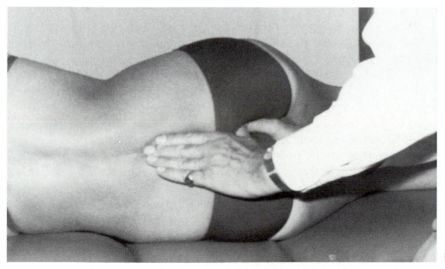

b

Fig. 7.5 (a) and **(b)** Treatment of inferior innominate shear.

part of her right ischial tuberosity and your index finger medial to her right posterior superior iliac spine.

(d) The patient should start forced inhalation and exhalation while you lift her right innominate and try to slide it craniad.

(e) Re-examine and repeat as necessary.

Lumbar spine

The next priority is the examination for maladaptive dysfunction in the lumbar and low thoracic spine. If this is found, it is treated before proceeding.

Sacral torsions

1. Anterior sacral torsion, left on left, diagnosis.
(a) Sitting FFT, positive right (usually).
(b) Sitting FFT for ILA (inferior lateral angle of sacrum), positive left. If this sign is positive, there is presumptive evidence of anterior torsion.
(c) ILA prone, left posterior. May become level in extension.
(d) Sacral base, anterior right.
(e) Lumbar lordosis, increased. Springing test negative.
(f) Medial malleolus prone, high left, because lumbar scoliosis convex right.
(g) Lumbar adaptation, L5 rotated right.
Anterior, left on left, sacral torsion, treatment (Fig. 7.6).
(a) The patient starts lying prone. Her right shoulder should be close to the edge of the table.
(b) You stand on her right and lift her legs so that you turn her pelvis to the right and bring up the knees so that they and her hips are at about a right angle. This is sometimes known as the left lateral Sims position (Fig. 7.6a).
(c) Monitor at L5–S1 with your right hand and use your left hand to flex her legs until the sacrum just begins to move. *Do not flex the lumbosacral joint.*
(d) She should breathe deeply and, on exhalation, reach for the floor with her right hand. Repeat until you feel the movement reach the L4–5 joint. *Do not rotate L5.* It may be necessary to change your monitoring hand so that you can enourage this movement with your right one.
(e) Monitor again at L5–S1 with your right hand and help her not to lose the rotation by pressing down on her shoulder with your elbow. Either proceed as in step (f) or as in step (g), in which case the monitoring and active hands are reversed.
(f) *Either* Support her knees by putting one of your knees underneath. The table edge would hurt, a pillow may be used instead (Fig. 7.6b).
(g) *Or* Maintain her position while you turn round and sit on the table close to her thighs. Abduct your left thigh so that you can support her knees on your left knee (Fig. 7.7).

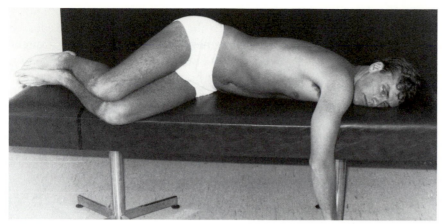

a

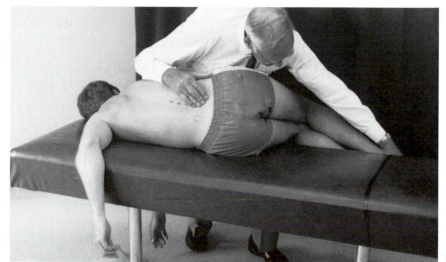

Fig. 7.6 (a) Left lateral Sims position. **(b)** Treatment of anterior sacral torsion (left on left).

b

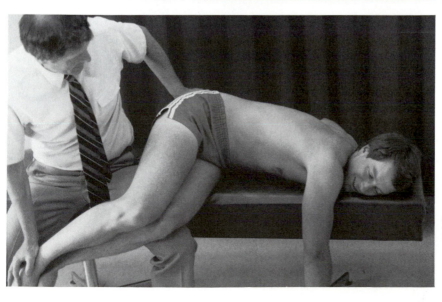

Fig. 7.7 Treatment of left on left torsion with operator sitting.

(h) She should drop her feet towards the floor as far as they will go.

(i) She attempts to raise her feet to the ceiling against the resistance of your left hand. Do not allow movement. When she does this it ought to be possible for you to feel the right side of the sacral base becoming more posterior.

(j) After 4 or 5 seconds, both relax, but do not lose the position. On full relaxation, take up the slack by following the descent of her feet with your hand.

(k) Repeat steps (h) and (i) three or four times.

(l) Re-examine.

2. Posterior, right on left, sacral torsion, diagnosis.

(a) Sitting FFT, positive right.

(b) ILA prone, right posterior worse on extension, level on flexion.

(c) Sacral base, anterior left.

(d) Lumbar lordosis, reduced and springing test positive.

(e) Medial malleolus prone, right high because the lumbar lordosis is convex left.

(f) Lumbar adaptation, L5 rotated left.

(g) *Note that the parameters for posterior torsion are the same as those for anterior torsion with the exception of the effect of lumbar flexion/extension (ILA movement, lumbar lordosis and springing test).*

Posterior, right on left, sacral torsion, treatment (Fig. 7.8).

(a) The patient lies on her left side near the front of the table.

(b) You stand facing her and rotate her upper trunk by pulling her left shoulder out from under her.

(c) Extend her left leg, allowing the right leg to lie in front of it, and

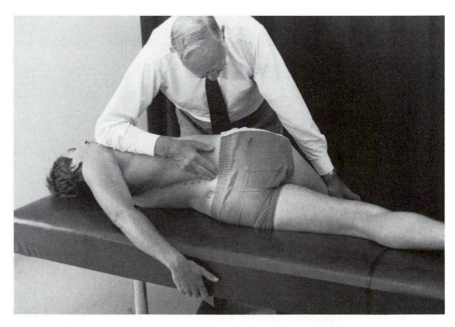

Fig. 7.8 Treatment of posterior sacral torsion (right on left).

then monitor with your right hand at her lumbosacral junction while you push her left leg backwards to extend her hip until movement reaches the sacrum but not L5.

(d) Monitor at L5–S1 with your left hand and have her breathe out while you rotate her right shoulder backwards. The object is to rotate the trunk to the right, down to L5 but not to S1. The movement will usually have to be repeated once or twice. When the position is correct, she should grip the far edge of the table with her right hand in order to maintain the position.

(e) Change hands again and drop her right leg over the side of the table. Place your left hand on the side of her right knee. Use your right hand to monitor at L5–S1.

(f) She should attempt to raise her right knee to the ceiling against your unyielding resistance. Hold the position for 4 or 5 seconds and then relax.

(g) On full relaxation, take up the slack by depression of her knee and repeat three or four times. The slack should be taken up until you feel the sacrum just begin to move.

(h) Re-examine.

3. Note that, in both the torsion techniques, the principle is to line up the lumbar spine with the sacrum in neutral flexion/extension at the L5–S1 joint and, by sidebending, force the sacrum to rotate according to 'neutral spinal mechanics'.

Sacral shears

1. Inferior sacral shear (unilateral sacral flexion) on the left, diagnosis.
(a) Sitting FFT, positive left.
(b) ILA prone, left inferior more than posterior, do not become level in flexion or extension.
(c) Sacral base, anterior left.
(d) Lumbar lordosis, normal or increased.
(e) Lumbar scoliosis, convex left.
(f) Medial malleolus prone, left low.
(g) Lumbar adaptation, sidebent right.
Inferior sacral shear left, treatment (Fig. 7.9).
(a) The patient lies prone.
(b) You stand beside her left hip.
(c) With your left hand, monitor in the sulcus medial to the PSIS.
(d) With your right hand, adjust the position of her left leg to bring her left sacroiliac joint to its point of maximum ease. (Loose-pack the joint.) This usually needs slight abduction and internal rotation of the thigh. Tell her to hold her leg in that position.
(e) Press downwards on her left ILA with the heel of your right hand. Try springing in varying directions until you find the one that produces most movement at your monitoring fingers. This is best done with a straight elbow.
(f) She should inhale deeply and hold it for several seconds while you keep up the pressure.

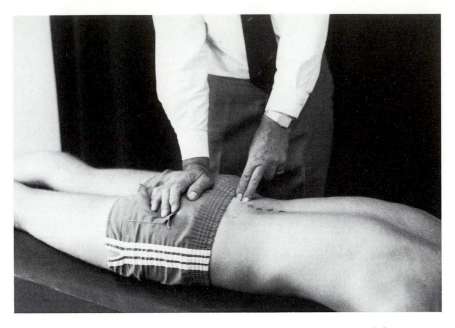

Fig. 7.9 Treatment of unilateral inferior sacral shear (sacral flexion) on the left.

(g) Maintain the pressure while she exhales slowly and then keep pressing while she repeats the cycle three or four times. Finally release the pressure slowly.

(h) Re-examine.

2. Superior sacral shear left, diagnosis.

(a) Sitting FFT, positive left.

(b) ILA prone, left superior and slightly anterior, do not become level in flexion or extension.

(c) Sacral base, posterior left.

(d) Lumbar lordosis, reduced.

(e) Lumbar scoliosis, convex right.

(f) Medial malleolus prone, high left.

(g) Lumbar adaptation, sidebent left.

Superior sacral shear left, treatment (Fig. 7.10).

(a) The patient lies prone in the sphinx position, to extend L5.

(b) You stand beside her right hip.

(c) Loose-pack her left sacroiliac joint by abduction. *Do not internally rotate the thigh; that would 'bind' the front of the sacroiliac joint.*

(d) Contact her left sacral base with your right pisiform and lift under her left ASIS with your left hand.

(e) Have her make a forced exhalation while you apply pressure with your pisiform and lift with your left hand.

(f) She should relax but keep the position and then repeat two or three times. This procedure is painful.

(g) Re-examine.

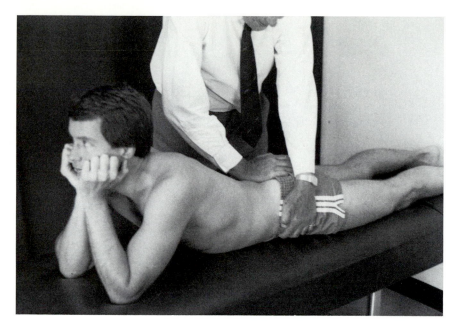

Fig. 7.10 Treatment of unilateral superior sacral shear (sacral extension) on the left.

3. Bilateral sacral shears. These are rare but can occur. The signs tend to be confusing because they are the same on the two sides. In a bilateral superior shear the lumbar lordosis will be lost, in the inferior shear it will be deep. The treatment is the same as for the unilateral shear but is repeated on the other side.

Innominate rotations

1. Posterior innominate on the left, diagnosis.
(a) Standing FFT, positive left.
(b) ASIS left, superior and slightly posterior.
(c) Sacral sulcus, left deep.
(d) PSIS left, posterior and slightly inferior.
(e) Medial malleolus supine, left high.
Posterior innominate on the left, treatment.
(a) Muscle energy prone, with high velocity variant (Fig. 7.11).
    (i) The patient is prone.
    (ii) You stand beside her right hip.
    (iii) With your left hand, lift her left leg just above the knee.
    (iv) Monitor with your right fingers in the left sulcus and move her left leg to loose-pack her sacroiliac joint. This usually requires slight abduction and rotation.
    (v) Place your right hand on her left iliac crest just in front of the PSIS.
    (vi) Lift her leg with your left hand to the barrier and take out

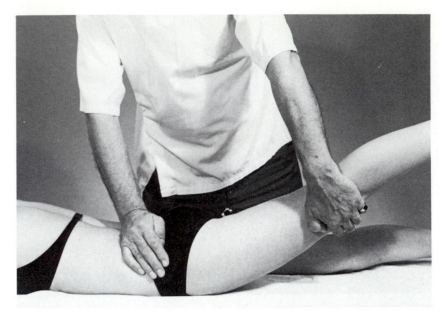

Fig. 7.11 Prone muscle energy treatment of left posterior innominate.

any slack by pressing down on her iliac crest. The sacrum should not have moved.

(vii) She should attempt to pull her leg down to the table while you resist. Maximum force is not needed, you must prevent movement.

(viii) Have her relax and, when she has done so fully, take up the slack by lifting her left leg to the new barrier.

(ix) Repeat steps (vii) and (viii) three or four times.

(x) *Or*, if you wish to use a thrust, instead of step (vii), give a high velocity low amplitude thrust downwards on the back of her iliac crest. At the same time you should increase the upward pull on her thigh as counterforce.

(xi) Re-examine.

(b) Muscle energy sidelying (Fig. 7.12).

(i) The patient lies on her right side.

(ii) You stand behind her hips and place your right hand against the back of her left iliac crest.

(iii) Have her lift her left leg with the knee bent to a right angle.

(iv) With your left hand, grasp her left ankle and pull gently towards you to take up the slack.

(v) Have her attempt to pull her knee forwards while you resist with forward pressure of your right hand and a backward pull with your left hand.

(vi) After 4 or 5 seconds, she should relax and, when she has done so fully, you take up the slack with your left hand.

(vii) Repeat steps (v) and (vi) three or four times and then re-examine.

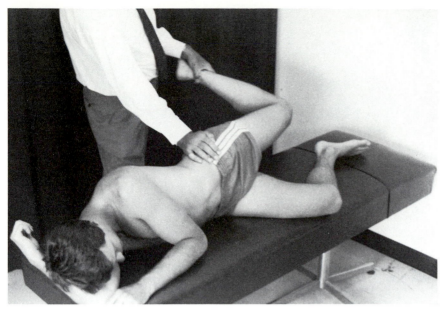

Fig. 7.12 Sidelying muscle energy treatment of left posterior innominate.

(viii) If preferred, this can be done with her knee straight. You then hold her left thigh just above the knee with your left hand.

(c) Muscle energy supine. This treatment is the same as that described earlier (see Fig. 7.1) for the superior pubis except that the patient is nearer the edge of the table. The sacrum should remain on the table but the PSIS should be just off the edge.

(d) High velocity sidelying (Fig. 7.13).

(i) The patient lies on her right side.

(ii) You stand in front of her thighs.

(iii) With your left hand, pull her right shoulder forwards (out from under) to rotate her spine to the left.

(iv) Bring her left knee over the edge of the table. You may wish her foot to hang free, or it can be tucked into the bend of her right knee.

(v) Use your left hand on the front of her left shoulder to complete the left rotation of her spine down to the sacrum.

(vi) Place your right pisiform in contact with the ledge under her left PSIS, with your forearm horizontal and making an angle of about 30° to the long axis of her body.

(vii) When you have taken up the slack, make a high velocity, low amplitude thrust with your right hand in the direction in which your forearm points. The pressure of your left hand on her shoulder will need to be slightly increased as counterforce.

(viii) If there is difficulty, it may help if you 'gap' the sacroiliac joint by pressing down on her left knee with your left knee as you do the thrust.

(ix) Re-examine.

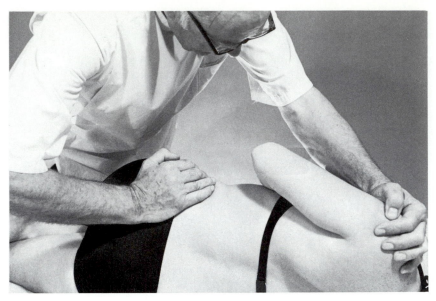

Fig. 7.13 Sidelying high velocity treatment of left posterior innominate.

2. Anterior innominate on the left, diagnosis.
(a) Standing FFT, positive left.
(b) ASIS, left low.
(c) Sacral sulcus, left shallow.
(d) PSIS, left anterior and slightly high.
(e) Medial malleolus supine, left low.
Anterior innominate on the left, treatment.
(a) Muscle energy sidelying (Fig. 7.14).
    (i) The patient lies on her right side.
    (ii) You stand in front of her hips.
    (iii) With your right hand, monitor for movement in her left sacral sulcus.
    (iv) With your left hand, bend up her left knee and hip until the innominate has begun to move but the sacrum has not.
    (v) Stand so that you can resist movement of her left leg with your hip or abdomen.
    (vi) She should try to straighten her left leg while you resist.
    (vii) After 4 or 5 seconds, she can relax and, when she has done so fully, take up the slack to the new barrier by further flexion of her left leg.
    (viii) Repeat steps (vi) and (vii) three or four times and then re-examine.
(b) High velocity, sidelying (Fig. 7.15).
    (i) The patient lies on her right side.
    (ii) You stand facing her hips.
    (iii) Position her right leg straight on the table.

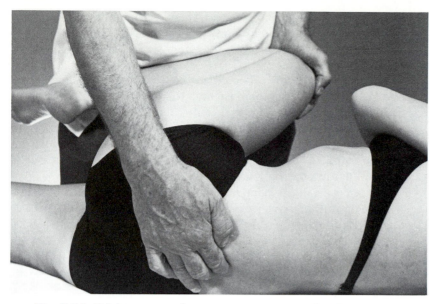

Fig. 7.14 Sidelying muscle energy treatment of right anterior innominate.

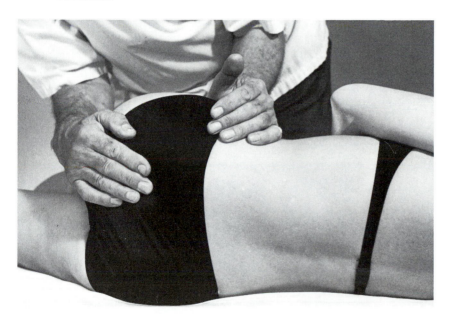

Fig. 7.15 Sidelying high velocity treatment of right anterior innominate.

(iv) Bend her left hip so that her leg hangs over the edge of the table.

(v) Grasp her left ischial tuberosity with your right hand and press back on the anterior end of her left iliac crest with your left hand.

(vi) Take up any slack and then give a high velocity, low

amplitude thrust forward with your right hand on her ischial tuberosity. Your left hand only slightly increases its pressure posteriorly on the crest.

(vii) Re-examine.

(c) Muscle energy supine, described for a right anterior innominate (Fig. 7.16). This is very similar to that for an inferior pubis (see Fig. 7.2), but note the differences.

(i) The patient lies supine with her right hip and knee fully flexed. You need to be able to resist the movement of her leg with your trunk. The usual method is to lean over her and put her right knee in your right axilla.

(ii) You stand on her left and slide your left hand under her buttock so that your index finger reaches the lateral side of her right PSIS and your middle finger is in the sulcus between the sacrum and ilium. You can then monitor to see that you do not flex her leg too far and 'bind' the sacroiliac joint.

(iii) With the palm of your left hand, pull on her ischial tuberosity in the direction of her right ASIS.

(iv) Press down on her right ASIS with your right hand.

(v) She should attempt to push her right foot towards the foot of the table, or simply 'try to push me away'. The force must be controlled or you will not be able to prevent movement.

(vi) Both relax but you maintain the position.

(vii) When she has fully relaxed you take up the slack by increasing the hip flexion. Monitor with your left hand and stop before the sacrum begins to move.

(viii) When you have reached the new barrier, repeat steps (v), (vi) and (vii) two or three times and then re-examine.

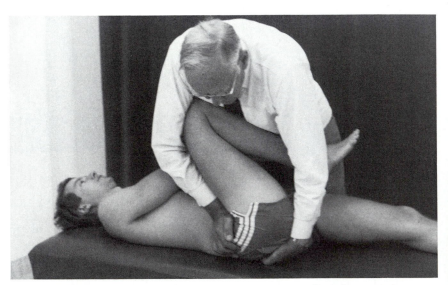

Fig. 7.16 Supine muscle energy treatment of right anterior innominate.

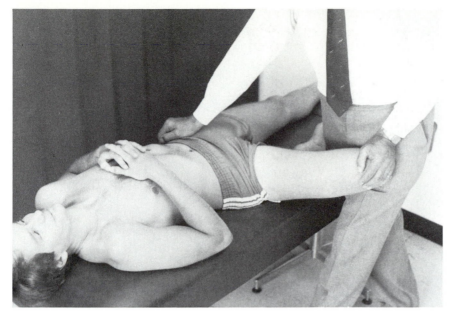

Fig. 7.17 Treatment of iliac inflare on the right.

Iliac flares

1. Iliac inflare on the right, diagnosis.
(a) Standing FFT, positive right.
(b) ASIS, medial right.
(c) PSIS, lateral right.
(d) Sacral sulcus, wide right.
Iliac inflare on the right, treatment (Fig. 7.17).
(a) The patient lies supine with her right hip fully flexed and abducted.
(b) You stand on her right.
(c) With your left hand, hold her right hip abducted and put your right hand on the medial aspect of her left ASIS.
(d) Have her make an adduction effort which you resist with an equal counterforce.
(e) After 4 or 5 seconds, both relax and, when she has fully relaxed, take up the slack to the new barrier.
(f) Repeat steps (e) and (f) three or four times and then re-examine.
2. Iliac outflare on the left, diagnosis.
(a) Standing FFT, positive left. *Note that the other parameters are the same for a right inflare.*
(b) ASIS, lateral left.
(c) PSIS, medial left.
(d) Sacral sulcus, narrow left.
Iliac outflare on the left, treatment (Fig. 7.18).
(a) The patient lies supine with her left hip fully flexed and adducted.
(b) You stand on her left side at hip level and lean across her so that, with your trunk, you can prevent abduction of her left hip.

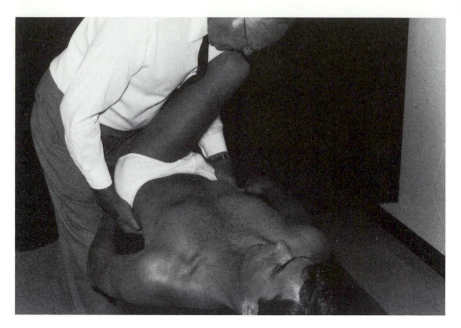

Fig. 7.18   Treatment of iliac outflare on the left.

(c) With your left hand, hold the lateral aspect of her right ilium, or reach under her and with your fingertips grasp her left PSIS and pull it towards you.

(d) Have her try to abduct her left leg by pushing towards you while you resist the movement.

(e) After 4 or 5 seconds, both relax and when she has relaxed fully, take up the slack by further adduction.

(f) Repeat steps (d) and (e) three or four times and then re-examine.

Chapter 8

Treatment of the Lumbar and Thoracic Spine, Fully Specific

PRINCIPLES

There is a very wide variety of techniques that have been described and almost all of them can be altered to suit the individual circumstances of treatment of a specific patient by a particular therapist. There are circumstances under which it is necessary to devise a different technique to deal with a special problem.

It is most important, therefore, that the principles should be well understood. The principles are the same, no matter if one is using a semispecific or a fully specific technique, nor do they change whether one uses a direct or indirect, or even an exaggeration method. The techniques described here will be direct action techniques where the barrier is engaged and either pushed away by *high velocity* or encouraged to recede by *muscle energy*.

The basic principles are as follows.

1. Examination to discover the exact level to be treated (see Chapter 5).

2. Examination to discover the precise location of the barrier and thus to determine the direction in which the joint needs to be treated (see Chapter 5).

3. Positioning the patient in such a way that the force used will be concentrated at the level intended (see Chapter 6).

4. Application of force that will result in at least partial removal of the barrier without damaging neighbouring structures.

5. In thrusting techniques the force must be sufficient to move the joint but not so much that it does damage. Dr John Mennell has said many times that the movement at the joint should be less than 'an eighth of an inch' (3 mm).

6. When muscle energy techniques are used for spinal joints, the force exerted by the patient must be restricted. Many of the muscles with which we are most concerned are small and relatively weak. If too much force is used, other muscles will be recruited and the specificity of the effort will be compromised. When first trying to do this, almost all patients tend to push too hard.

7. In many techniques the patient can be treated by either muscle energy or high velocity thrusting from the same position. In both, the

essential requirement is that the joint barrier should be lightly engaged in all three planes.

There are significant differences in the methods used for diagnosis and treatment between the specific and the semispecific techniques. There is little doubt that the fully specific techniques are the more accurate and the authors do not advise the use of muscle energy treatment techniques unless a full specific diagnosis has been made.

THE LUMBAR SPINE

Sidelying techniques

The first three techniques can be used for high velocity thrusting, for muscle energy or even for articulatory treatment. They are basically similar and, in each, the patient lies on the side of the most posterior transverse process. There are many possible variants. The movement used to perform the thrusting manipulations is rotatory and it must be remembered that the range of rotation in the lumbar joints is very small. The effort used in the muscle energy techniques may be rotatory or, in the later examples, sidebending.

These techniques all use *long levers*, the forces being applied at a distance from the joint. Localisation depends on precise positioning of the structures on both sides of the joint to be treated. A variant for high velocity treatment using a short lever on the caudal side is described in the note after the third technique (see p. 125); it can be applied to any of the first three. If, for any reason, localisation by the described method proves to be difficult, the hybrid technique using one long and one short lever may be easier.

Technique 1a

For non-neutral, type II dysfunction with restriction of flexion and of sidebending and rotation to the left (ERS$_R$) described for L3–4 (Fig. 8.1).

1. Diagnostic points.
    (a) With the patient prone, the right transverse process of L3 is slightly more prominent (posterior) than the left.
    (b) With the patient flexed, the right transverse process of L3 is more posterior.
    (c) With the patient extended (in the sphinx position), the transverse processes of L3 are nearly or completely level.
2. Treatment.
    (a) The patient lies on her right side with her head supported by a pillow or by her arm. Ease her shoulders slightly forward to flex her upper spine. This position on a table causes the spine to bend slightly to the left. Do not pull her right shoulder out from under her, that would produce an unwanted right sidebend.
    (b) You stand at the side of the table facing her.

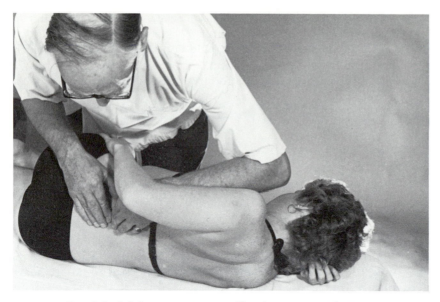

Fig. 8.1 Sidelying treatment of lumbar spine with ERS_R.

(c) Monitor with your right hand while you ease her right shoulder forward enough to bring the tension down to L3.

(d) Thread your left arm through her left axilla and monitor movement with your left hand at the L3–4–5 interspaces.

(e) Use your right hand to drop her left leg over the front edge of the table and bring her right leg up behind it until you feel the tension begin to rise at the L4–5 space. Her right foot should remain on the table.

(f) Position your right forearm so that you can use your fingers to assist the monitoring at L3–4–5 and so that the forearm rests on her left buttock midway between the ASIS and the ischial tuberosity.

(g) 'Fine tune' the position by rotation. Use your right forearm to rotate her left buttock forwards and your left forearm on the front of her left shoulder to rotate her upper trunk backwards. The end-point (when you reach the barrier) is when the tension in the tissues just reaches L3 from above and L4 from below.

(h) High velocity variant.

    (i) Make sure that the patient is relaxed. If she is not, a few deep breaths in and out will sometimes help. Be sure after this that you are still at the barrier (it may have moved).

    (ii) Apply a short sharp thrust equally with your right forearm forward on her buttock and with your left forearm backward on her shoulder.

(i) Muscle energy variant.

    (i) Move your right hand to the lateral aspect of her left knee.

    (ii) Ask her to attempt to raise her left knee toward the ceiling while you resist with an equal and opposite force and with counterforce on the front of her left shoulder.

(iii) After 4 or 5 seconds both relax, but do not lose your position.

(iv) When she has relaxed fully you take up the slack (to the new barrier) by further rotation.

(v) Repeat steps (ii), (iii) and (iv) three or four times.

(j) Retest.

Technique 1b

For non-neutral, type II dysfunction with restriction of extension and of sidebending and rotation to the left (FRS$_R$), described for L3–4 (Fig. 8.2).

1. Diagnostic points.

(a) With the patient prone, the right transverse process of L3 is slightly more prominent (posterior) than the left.

(b) With the patient flexed, the transverse processes of L3 are nearly or completely level.

(c) With the patient extended (in the sphinx position), the right transverse process of L3 is more posterior.

2. Treatment.

(a) The patient lies on her right side with her head supported by a pillow or by her arm. This position on a table causes the spine to bend slightly to the left. Do not pull her right shoulder out from under her as that would produce an unwanted right sidebend.

(b) You stand at the side of the table facing her. Make sure that she is relaxed while you pull her L3–4 level towards you to start extension of the spine.

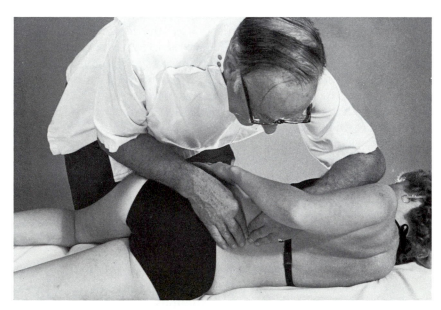

Fig. 8.2 Sidelying treatment of lumbar spine with FRS$_R$.

(c) Monitor at the L3–4 level with your right hand while you adjust the extension from above by pushing her right shoulder back until the tension begins to rise at the L2–3 level.

(d) Thread your left arm through her left axilla and monitor movement with your left hand at the L3–4–5 interspaces.

(e) Adjust the extension from below by pushing her right leg back until the tension begins to rise at the L4–5 level.

(f) Bring her left leg forward and allow it to hang over the front of the table.

(g) Position your right forearm so that you can use your fingers to assist the monitoring at L3–4–5 and so that the forearm rests on her left buttock midway between the ASIS and the ischial tuberosity.

(h) 'Fine tune' the rotation by using your right forearm to rotate her left buttock forwards and your left forearm on the front of her left shoulder to rotate her upper trunk backwards. The end-point (when you reach the barrier) is when the tension in the tissues just reaches L3 from above and L4 from below.

(i) High velocity variant.

> (i) Make sure that the patient is relaxed. If she is not, a few deep breaths in and out will sometimes help. Be sure after this that you are still at the barrier (it may have moved).

> (ii) Apply a short sharp thrust equally with your right forearm forward on her buttock and with your left forearm backward on her shoulder.

(j) Muscle energy variant.

> (i) Move your right hand to the lateral aspect of her left knee.

> (ii) Ask her to attempt to raise her left knee toward the ceiling while you resist with an equal and opposite force and with counterforce on the front of her left shoulder.

> (iii) After 4 or 5 seconds both relax, but do not lose your position.

> (iv) When she has relaxed fully you take up the slack (to the new barrier) by further rotation.

> (v) Repeat steps (ii), (iii) and (iv) three or four times.

(k) Retest.

Technique 1c

For neutral, type I dysfunction with the convexity to the right side (N_R) (restriction of sidebending to the right and rotation to the left), described for L2, 3 and 4 (Fig. 8.3).

1. Diagnostic points.

(a) With the patient prone, L2, 3 and 4 are rotated to the right (right transverse processes posterior). The amount of rotation is greater at L3 than at L4 and correspondingly at L2 than at L3, i.e. at each level there is rotation as compared to the bone below.

(b) With the patient either flexed or extended, a right rotation of the three vertebrae remains although it may alter in degree.

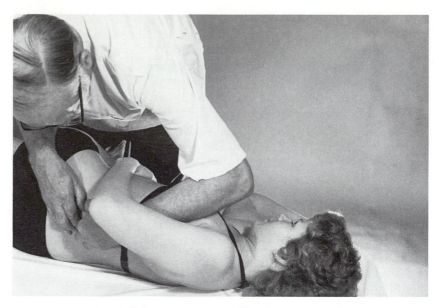

Fig. 8.3 Sidelying treatment of lumbar spine with N_R.

2. Treatment.

(a) The patient lies on her right side. In neutral dysfunctions the sidebend restriction is to the side opposite to that of the rotation. For this reason you do not support the head but you pull her right shoulder forwards so that her head lies on the table top. This produces a slight sidebend to the right.

(b) You stand at the side of the table facing her. Do not either flex or extend her spine.

(c) Thread your left arm through her left axilla and monitor movement with your left hand at the L3-4-5 interspaces.

(d) Flex her left knee and hip until you begin to feel movement at the L4–5 interspace.

(e) Position your right forearm so that you can use your fingers to assist the monitoring at L2–3–4–5 and so that the forearm rests on her left buttock midway between the ASIS and the ischial tuberosity.

(f) 'Fine tune' the position by using your right forearm to rotate her left buttock forwards and your left forearm on the front of her left shoulder to rotate her upper trunk backwards. The end-point (when you reach the barrier) is when the tension in the tissues just reaches L3 from above and L4 from below.

(g) High velocity variant.

   (i) Make sure that the patient is relaxed. If she is not, a few deep breaths in and out will sometimes help. Be sure after this that you are still at the barrier (it may have moved).

   (ii) Apply a short sharp thrust equally with your right forearm forward on her buttock and with your left forearm backward on her shoulder.

(h) Muscle energy variant.

    (i) Move your right hand to the lateral aspect of her left knee.

    (ii) Ask her to attempt to raise her left knee toward the ceiling while you resist with an equal and opposite force and with counterforce on the front of her left shoulder.

    (iii) After 4 or 5 seconds both relax, but do not lose your position.

    (iv) When she has relaxed fully you take up the slack (to the new barrier) by further rotation.

    (v) Repeat steps (ii), (iii) and (iv) three or four times.

(i) Retest.

Note. For any of the first three techniques there is a variant using a short lever for the caudal side of the joint to be treated.

1. Steps 1(e), 2(h) and 3(e) would be changed to read (in each case): 'Position your right pisiform bone so that it is directly behind and touching the left transverse process of her L4 vertebra.'

2. 'Lean over the patient enough so that your right forearm can extend horizontally backwards behind her. The thrust is given by a *short* sharp movement of your right forearm forwards with a controlling backward pressure on her left shoulder.'

Alternative sidelying techniques

These are all long lever techniques for which accurate localisation is important.

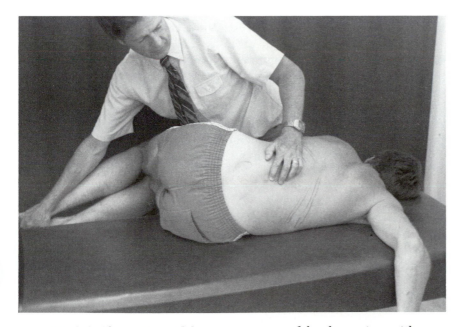

Fig. 8.4 Alternative sidelying treatment of lumbar spine with ERS_L. For the variant with the operator sitting, compare Fig. 7.7.

Technique 2

For restriction of flexion. This is a muscle energy treatment for type II dysfunction. Described for restriction of sidebending and rotation to the right (ERS$_L$), at L3–4 (Fig. 8.4).

   1. Diagnostic points.

   (a) With the patient prone, the left transverse process of L3 is slightly more prominent (posterior) than the right.

   (b) With the patient flexed, the left transverse process of L3 is more posterior.

   (c) With the patient extended (in the sphinx position), the transverse processes of L3 are nearly or completely level.

   2. Treatment.

   (a) The patient lies in the lateral 'Sims' position on her right side (the side of the convexity in the lumbar spine). That is, she has her pelvis lying on the right side and the upper trunk prone. This position rotates the top to the right and also sidebends to the right.

   (b) You stand facing her abdomen and flex both her hips and knees to about a right angle. If you use the standing position, it is kind to have a pad between her thighs and the edge of the table or to be ready to support her thighs with your left knee. See step (f) for the alternative position of the operator.

   (c) Monitor with your right hand while you press down on her left shoulder to bring the rotation movement down to L3. If necessary, she can help by reaching for the floor with her left hand at the end of a deep exhalation and this may be repeated.

   (d) Flex her legs until the tension reaches L4.

   (e) *Either* monitor with your left hand and drop her feet off the edge of the table. This produces the necessary sidebend of L3 on L4.

   (f) *Or* sit on the edge of the table close to her thighs. Abduct your right thigh so that you can support her knees with your right knee and proceed using your left hand to resist her movement and your right hand to monitor.

   (g) Ask her to attempt to lift her feet towards the ceiling while you resist with your right hand. If the position is correct, you should feel the muscle tighten on the left side of the L3–4 joint.

   (h) After 4 or 5 seconds both relax, but do not lose the position. When she has relaxed fully, take up the slack by dropping the feet a little more.

   (i) Repeat steps (f) and (g) three or four times.

   (j) Retest.

Technique 3

This is a muscle energy treatment for a type II dysfunction with restriction of extension and of sidebending and rotation to the right (FRS$_L$), described for L3–4 (Fig. 8.5).

   1. Diagnostic points.

   (a) With the patient prone, the left transverse process of L3 is slightly more prominent (posterior) than the right.

(b) With the patient flexed, the transverse processes of L3 are nearly or completely level.

(c) With the patient extended (in the sphinx position), the left transverse process of L3 is more posterior.

2. Treatment.

(a) The patient lies on her left side.

(b) You stand at the side of the table facing her.

(c) Pull her L3–4 level towards you to induce extension. This must be a passive movement.

(d) Monitor on the left side of L3–4 with your free hand.

(e) Fine tune her position from above by pushing her left shoulder back.

(f) Fine tune from below by pushing her left leg back.

(g) Ask her to reach down with her right hand and hold the edge of the table behind her. The reaching down induces right sidebending, the reaching back for the table edge induces rotation.

(h) Lift her right foot with the knee bent until you feel the tension with your monitoring hand.

(i) Ask her to attempt to pull it down to her left knee. You should feel the contraction at L3.

(j) After 4 or 5 seconds both relax, and when she has relaxed fully, lift her right foot to the new barrier.

(k) Repeat steps (i) and (j) three or four times.

(l) Retest.

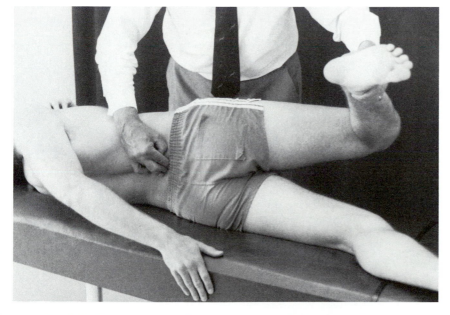

Fig. 8.5 Alternative sidelying treatment of lumbar spine with FRS_L.

Technique 4

This is a muscle energy treatment for neutral, type I dysfunction with the convexity to the right side (N_R) (restriction of sidebending to the right and of rotation to the left), described for L2, 3 and 4 (Fig. 8.6).

    1. Diagnostic points.
    (a) With the patient prone, L2, 3 and 4 are rotated to the right (right transverse processes posterior).
    (b) With the patient either flexed or extended, a right rotation of the three vertebrae remains although it may alter in degree.
    2. Treatment.
    (a) The patient lies on her left side.
    (b) You stand at the side of the table facing her.
    (c) Monitor with your right hand at L2–3–4.
    (d) Bend up her hips and knees until you reach the 'point of ease' at the middle of the group (L3), i.e. *when the tension is at a minimum.*
    (e) Lift her feet towards the ceiling until you feel movement at L4.
    (f) Ask her to attempt to pull her feet down against your resistance.
    (g) After 4 or 5 seconds both relax, and when she has relaxed fully, take up the slack by a further lift of her feet.
    (h) Repeat steps (f) and (g) three or four times.
    (i) Retest.

Sitting techniques

The three techniques to be described under this heading can be used for high velocity, muscle energy or articulatory treatment, but is is diffi-

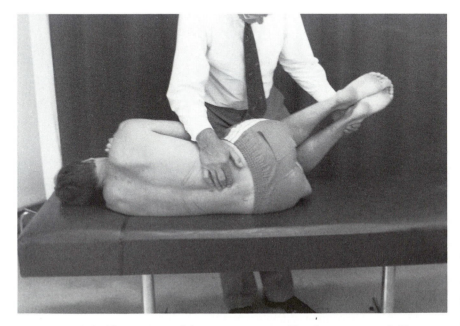

Fig. 8.6 Alternative sidelying treatment of lumbar spine with N_R.

cult to use them for high velocity treatment at L5–S1 and rather difficult at L4–5. With that warning, the sitting techniques are often much easier for a small person treating a large patient.

These techniques are also applicable to the lower thoracic joints and can be used conveniently up to T6 or even T5.

It is possible to use either hand as monitor; the descriptions will assume that the left hand is being so used. It is easier, for the technique described below, to use as monitor your hand of the side on which the transverse process is posterior.

The concept of obtaining both forward or backward and sidebending movement by *translation* will be introduced. This method has two great advantages: it keeps the patient's centre of gravity over her seat, and the movement is simultaneously introduced both above and below the joint.

These are long lever techniques requiring accurate localisation from above, but reliance is placed on the weight of the patient to stabilise the bone below the dysfunction.

Technique 5a

For restriction of flexion. Described for a type II dysfunction with restriction of sidebending and rotation to the right (ERS_L) at L1-2 (Fig. 8.7 in which, in order to show the patient's position, the operator is holding himself away; for actual treatment he would support the patient with his trunk).

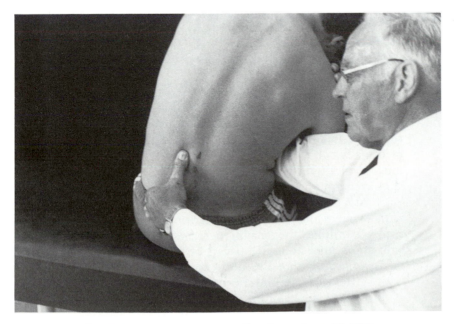

Fig. 8.7 Sitting treatment of lumbar spine with ERS_L.

1. Diagnostic points.

(a) With the patient prone, the left transverse process of L1 is slightly more prominent (posterior) than the right.

(b) With the patient flexed, the left transverse process of L1 is more posterior.

(c) With the patient extended (in the sphinx position) the transverse processes of L1 are nearly or completely level.

2. Treatment.

(a) The patient sits on a stool or with her legs over the side of the table or she may sit astride the table with her back at one end.

(b) You stand or sit behind her.

(c) Ask her to 'sit up tall' (any slump will restrict motion) and grasp her right shoulder with her left hand.

(d) Pass your right hand through her right axilla, across the front of her chest, and grasp her left humerus. Stand close enough so that you can pull her right shoulder against your chest to improve control. (There are a variety of different grips that can be used instead.)

(e) Monitor with your left thumb over the left transverse process of L1. If preferred, the thumb, or the base of the thenar eminence, may contact and monitor there or on the right side of the spinous process of L1.

(f) Ask her to slump so that L1 is translated backwards to introduce flexion from both above and below. This movement must be controlled and stopped as soon as the tension begins to build on either side of the joint.

(g) Translate her L1 level to the left to introduce right sidebending while you monitor your left thumb.

(h) With your right hand and trunk, rotate her trunk to the right until you feel the tension begin to accumulate at the L1 level. You have now engaged the barrier in all three planes.

(i) High velocity variant.

(i) Bring your left hip up behind your left elbow to increase your control.

(ii) With your thumb (or the base of your thenar eminence) on the left transverse process or the right side of the spinous process of L1, give a short sharp thrust to produce right rotation and right sidebending of L1 on L2. Sidebending is more easily obtained by thrusting on the spinous process. While the thrust is given, you must maintain the flexion.

(j) Muscle energy variant.

(i) Ask her to attempt to sidebend to her left while you resist with an equal and opposite counterforce. If the localisation is correct, you will feel the tension increase at the L1-2 level. An extension effort may be used instead of sidebending; rotation could be used but it is more difficult to control.

(ii) After 4 or 5 seconds both relax, but do not lose the position.

(iii) When she has relaxed fully, take up the slack in all three planes until you reach the new barrier.

(iv) Repeat steps (i), (ii) and (iii) three or four times.
(k) Retest.

Technique 5b

For restriction of extension. Described for a type II dysfunction with restriction of sidebending and rotation to the right (FRS$_L$) at L1–2 (Fig. 8.8 in which, in order to show the patient's position, the operator is holding himself away; for actual treatment he would support the patient with his trunk).

1. Diagnostic points.
(a) With the patient prone, the left transverse process of L1 is slightly more prominent (posterior) than the right.
(b) With the patient flexed, the transverse processes of L1 are nearly or completely level.
(c) With the patient extended (in the sphinx position), the left transverse process of L1 is more posterior.

2. Treatment.
(a) The patient sits on a stool or with her legs over the side of the table or she may sit astride the table with her back at one end.
(b) You stand or sit behind her.
(c) Ask her to 'sit up tall' (any slump will restrict motion) and grasp her right shoulder with her left hand.
(d) Pass your right hand through her right axilla, across the front of her chest, and grasp her left humerus. Stand close enough so that you can pull her right shoulder against your chest to improve control. (There is a variety of different grips that can be used instead.)

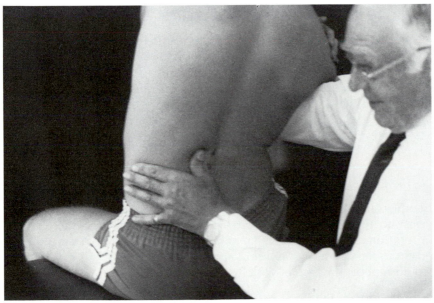

Fig. 8.8 Sitting treatment of lumbar spine with FRS$_L$.

(e) Monitor with your left thumb over the left transverse process of L1. If preferred, the thumb, or the base of the thenar eminence, may contact and monitor there or on the right side of the spinous process of L1.

(f) With your right hand and trunk, rotate her trunk to the right until you feel the tension begin to accumulate at the L1 level. Observe that the order of the movements is changed. Rotation is started first to make extension easier at the facet joint.

(g) Ask her to let you arch her back, which you do by translating L1 forwards to introduce extension from both above and below. This movement must be controlled and stopped as soon as the tension begins to build on either side of the joint.

(h) Translate her L1 level to the left to introduce right sidebending while you monitor with your left thumb.

(i) Check the rotation position and adjust if necessary. You have now engaged the barrier in all three planes.

(j) High velocity variant.

(i) Bring your left hip up behind your left elbow to increase your control.

(ii) With your thumb (or the base of your thenar eminence) on the left transverse process or the right side of the spinous process of L1, give a short sharp thrust to produce right rotation and right sidebending of L1 on L2. Sidebending is more easily obtained by thrusting on the spinous process. While the thrust is given, you must maintain the extension.

(k) Muscle energy variant.

(i) Ask her to attempt to sidebend to her left while you resist with an equal and opposite counterforce. If the localisation is correct, you will feel the tension increase at the L1–2 level. Sometimes it may be more effective to have the patient attempt to flex against your resistance. A rotatory effort can be used but it is more difficult for the operator to control the movement.

(ii) After 4 or 5 seconds both relax, but do not lose the position.

(iii) When she has relaxed fully, take up the slack in all three planes until you reach the new barrier.

(iv) Repeat steps (i), (ii) and (iii) three or four times.

(l) Retest.

Technique 5c

For neutral, type I dysfunction. Described for T12–L1–L2 with the convexity to the left side (N$_L$) (restriction of sidebending to the left and of rotation to the right) (Fig. 8.9 in which, in order to show the patient's position, the operator is holding himself away. For actual treatment he would support the patient with his trunk).

1. Diagnostic points.

(a) With the patient prone, T12, L1 and 2 are rotated to the left (left transverse processes posterior).

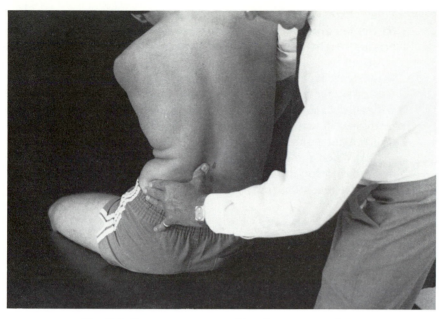

Fig. 8.9 Sitting treatment of lumbar spine with N$_L$.

(b) With the patient either flexed or extended, a left rotation of the three vertebrae remains although it may alter in degree.

2. Treatment.

(a) The patient sits on a stool or with her legs over the side of the table or she may sit astride the table with her back at one end.

(b) You stand or sit behind her.

(c) Ask her to 'sit up tall' (any slump will restrict motion) and grasp her right shoulder with her left hand.

(d) Pass your right hand through her right axilla, across the front of her chest, and grasp her left humerus. Stand close enough so that you can pull her right shoulder against your chest to improve control. (There is a variety of different grips that can be used instead.)

(e) Monitor with your left thumb over the left transverse process of L1. If preferred, the thumb, or the base of the thenar eminence, may contact and monitor there or on the right side of the spinous process of L1.

(f) With your right hand and trunk, rotate her trunk to the right until you feel the tension begin to accumulate at the L1 level.

(g) Translate her L1 level to the right to introduce left sidebending while you monitor with your left thumb.

(h) Do not either flex or extend to find a barrier, but a small adjustment of the sagittal plane position may sometimes be helpful in obtaining good localisation.

(i) High velocity variant.

    (i) Bring your left hip up behind your left elbow to increase your control.

(ii) With your thumb (or the base of your thenar eminence) on the left transverse process of L1, give a short sharp thrust to produce right rotation while you maintain the left sidebent position.

(j) Muscle energy variant.

(i) Ask her to attempt to sidebend to her right while you resist with an equal and opposite counterforce. If the localisation is correct you will feel the tension increase at the L1–2 level.

(ii) After 4 or 5 seconds both relax, but do not lose the position.

(iii) When she has relaxed fully, take up the slack in sidebending and rotation until you reach the new barrier.

(iv) Repeat steps (i), (ii) and (iii) three or four times.

(k) Retest.

THE LOWER THORACIC SPINE

It is possible in some patients to use the first three of the lumbar sidelying techniques for the lowest thoracic joints. With this type of technique, the amount of movement needed to change the localisation from one joint to the next at this level is small and one's ability to localise accurately improves a lot with practice. It is never easy to use one of these sidelying techniques above T9.

The sitting techniques described for the lumbar spine (numbers 5a, b and c) work well in the thoracic spine up to T5; above that level a different hold is necessary in order to control the patient's position and motion as is required.

Alternative high velocity techniques

Three additional high velocity techniques for the lower half of the thoracic spine will be described as well as both muscle energy and a variety of high velocity methods for the upper half. The high velocity techniques described for the upper thoracic spine numbers 10a, b and c can also be used down to T8 or 9 in most patients.

Technique 6

Supine treatment of lower thoracic dysfunction. These are hybrid techniques using a short lever (the transverse process) below and a long lever above. Accurate localisation from above is essential; the contact below is on the vertebra itself and localisation is automatic but correct positioning is a help in obtaining proper correction. They can be used up to T5.

Technique 6a

For restriction of flexion. Described for restriction of left rotation and sidebending at T8–9 (ERS$_R$) (Fig. 8.10).

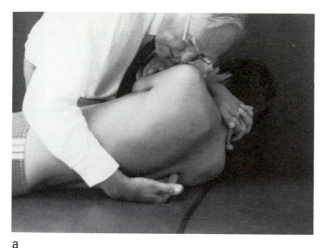
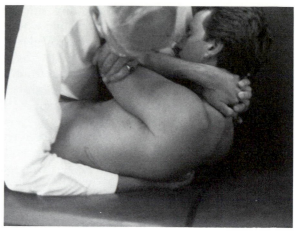

a

b

Fig. 8.10 Supine treatment of lower thoracic spine **(a)** to show hand placement, **(b)** for ERS$_R$.

1. Diagnostic points. These are the findings on dynamic examination. Compare the static findings for the similar lesion in technique 1a.

(a) In the erect position, the right transverse process of T8 is slightly more prominent than the left.

(b) On flexion, the right transverse process of T8 does not rise up and it becomes relatively more prominent.

(c) On extension, the transverse processes of T8 become level.

2. Treatment.

(a) The patient lies on her back.

(b) You stand on her right, you could do it from the left but it is usually easier if you are on the side of the most posterior transverse process (the side to which T8 is rotated).

(c) Ask her to lace her fingers together behind the base of her neck. It is important that the hands should be as low as possible, otherwise the head and neck become uncomfortably flexed which makes relaxation difficult.

(d) Lift her left shoulder with your left hand until you can get your right hand under her at the level to be treated. Your right hand should be held so that it can support the transverse processes on either side at the vertebra below the joint to be treated. This is best accomplished by flexing the interphalangeal joints but leaving the meta-carpophalangeal joints extended. The patient's spinous processes are then cradled in the groove, and the base of your thenar eminence should support the left transverse process of T9.

(e) Allow her shoulder to return to the table top with your hand under her.

(f) With your left hand, flex her upper back by using her elbows as levers. It is this movement that begins the localisation and it must be monitored by the tension in the paraspinal tissues as felt by your right hand.

(g) With your left hand on her elbows, you can both rotate her upper trunk and sidebend it as desired. In this example the rotation and sidebending would be to the left. This movement also must be monitored and controlled to bring the tension just to the level to be treated.

(h) When the barrier has been engaged in all three planes, with flexion/extension adjustment if necessary, you lean over so that you can press down on her elbows with your chest. The thrust is then given by a short sharp increase in that pressure with your body in the direction of the base of your right thenar eminence.

(i) While this technique is primarily for high velocity thrust treatment, it would be possible to use muscle energy activation by, for instance, having her attempt to extend against your resistance.

Technique 6b

For restriction of extension. Described for restriction of left rotation and sidebending at T8–9 (FRS$_R$) (Fig. 8.11).

1. Diagnostic points. These are the findings on dynamic examination. Compare the static findings for the similar lesion in technique 1b.

(a) In the erect position, the right transverse process of T8 is slightly more prominent than the left.

(b) On flexion, the transverse processes of T8 become level.

(c) On extension, the left transverse process of T8 does not come back down and the right process becomes more prominent.

2. Treatment.

Steps (a) to (g) are as for the flexion restricted lesion.

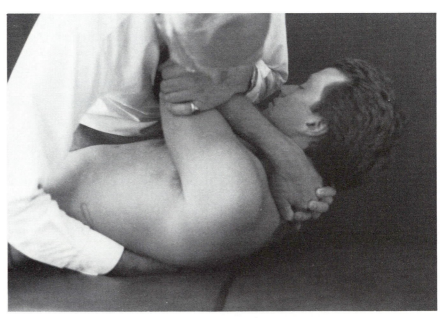

Fig. 8.11 Supine treatment of lower thoracic spine for FRS$_R$. For a neutral dysfunction, the picture would appear similar. For details of position see text.

(h) Allow her upper trunk to extend over your right hand just enough to take the tension off the T8 level altogether. Her spine will then be extended over your right hand.

(i) The thrust is given as before in the direction of the base of your right thenar eminence, but, because of the different position, a small pillow may be used over her elbows to protect the front of your chest.

Technique 6c

For neutral dysfunction. Described for restriction of right sidebending and of left rotation at T7–8–9–10 (N_R) (see Fig. 8.11).

1. Diagnostic points.
(a) In the erect position, the right transverse processes of T7, 8 and 9 are slightly more prominent than the left.
(b) In either flexion or extension, some rotation of the transverse processes of T7, 8 and 9 remains.
2. Treatment.
Steps (a) to (f) as in the treatment for flexion restriction.
(g) With your left hand on her elbows you can both rotate her upper trunk and sidebend it as desired. In this example, the rotation would be to the left and the sidebending to the right. This movement also must be monitored and controlled to bring the tension just to the level to be treated.
(h) In this variant also any excess flexion should be taken out by allowing partial extension over your hand.
(i) The thrust is given as before in the direction of your right thenar eminence.

Technique 7 ('crossed pisiform')

This is a prone technique for treatment of dysfunctions with restriction of extension (FRS lesions). It can be used anywhere from about T12 up to T4. It is a short lever technique and, although this makes localisation automatic, it means that great care must be taken to ensure that the force is stopped almost as soon as it starts. 'The movement at the joint is less than an eighth of an inch' (3 mm). Attention to the detail of the technique is important as, if performed carelessly, the costovertebral joints can be damaged. Described for T6 with restriction of extension and of rotation and sidebending to the left (FRS_R) (Fig. 8.12).

1. Diagnostic points.
(a) With the patient prone, the right transverse process of T6 is slightly more prominent (posterior) than the left.
(b) With the patient flexed, the transverse processes of T6 are nearly or completely level. Dynamically the right transverse process goes forward to be level with the left.
(c) With the patient extended (in the sphinx position), the right transverse process of T6 is more posterior. Dynamically the left transverse process does not come down and back.

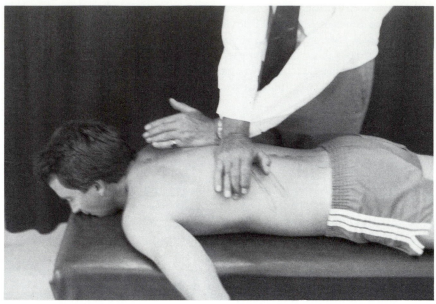

Fig. 8.12 Prone treatment of thoracic spine with FRS$_R$, the 'crossed pisiform' technique.

2. Treatment.

(a) The patient lies prone, perferably with her nose and chin accommodated by a slot in the table.

(b) You stand on the side of the most posterior transverse process (the right side in this example).

(c) Bring your left pisiform bone into contact with the caudal aspect of the right transverse process of her T6.

(d) Cross your hands to bring your right pisiform against the posterior surface of the left transverse process of T7.

(e) Ask her to inhale, to produce some extension of the spine.

(f) Give a *very short* sharp thrust with both hands simultaneously. The direction of the thrust is important. With your right hand it should be anterior and slightly craniad, with your left hand it should be craniad and only slightly anterior.

(g) Retest.

'Knee-in-back' techniques

These are sitting techniques of which there are many variants. They are basically semispecific, but can be adapted to be specific. The variations allow for their use with neutral or non-neutral dysfunctions.

Technique 8a

Sitting technique for restriction of extension in the lower thoracic spine with restriction of left rotation and left sidebending at T6–7 (FRS$_R$) (Fig. 8.13).

1. Diagnostic points.

(a) With the patient erect, the right transverse process of T6 is slightly more prominent (posterior) than the left.

(b) When the patient flexes, the right transverse process of T6 goes forward to be level with the left.

(c) When the patient extends, the left transverse process does not come down and back.

2. Treatment.

(a) The patient sits on a stool or with her legs over the side of the table.

(b) You stand behind her and you may need a stool with cross bars or some other support that will enable you to rest your foot at the required height. (Sometimes it is possible to use the table itself.)

(c) Ask her to lace her fingers behind the base of her neck with her elbows forward.

(d) Introduce your right hand through her right axilla and grip her right wrist. While adjusting her position, you use your left hand to monitor tension at T6–7.

(e) Place your left foot on a support of such a height that it will allow you to rest the front of your left knee against the back of the left transverse process of T7. Using your left knee to control the movement, translate T6–7 forward to induce extension.

(f) With your right hand, rotate her upper trunk to the left and sidebend her to the left at the same time. This and the previous movement must be controlled so that the tension is brought to the T6 level.

(g) Maintain the patient's position but insert your left hand through

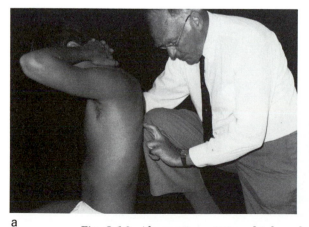
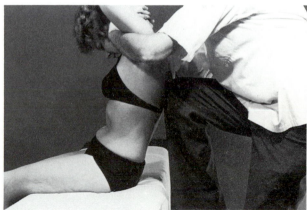

a
b

Fig. 8.13 Alternative sitting high velocity treatment for thoracic spine for FRS$_R$: **(a)** positioning the patient, **(b)** position before thrust. (See text for position to treat N$_R$ lesion.)

her left axilla and grip her left wrist. The operator's hand position can be seen in Fig. 9.6b (p. 159).

(h) Ask her to inhale to help extension and give a sharp pull posteriorly with both hands. This will extend and rotate T6 to the left with some sidebending.

Technique 8b

Sitting technique for restriction of flexion in the lower thoracic spine with restriction of left rotation and left sidebending at T6–7 (ERS$_R$) (Fig. 8.14, which shows an alternative position for the operator's hands).

1. Diagnostic points.

(a) With the patient erect, the right transverse process of T6 is slightly more prominent (posterior) than the left.

(b) When the patient flexes, the right transverse process of T6 does not go forward and the left becomes relatively higher and less prominent.

(c) When the patient extends, the left transverse process comes down and back to be level with the right.

2. Treatment.

(a) The patient sits on a stool or with her legs over the side of the table.

(b) You stand behind her and you may need a stool with cross bars or some other support that will enable you to rest your foot at the required height. (Sometimes it is possible to use the table itself.)

(c) Ask her to lace her fingers behind the base of her neck with her elbows forward.

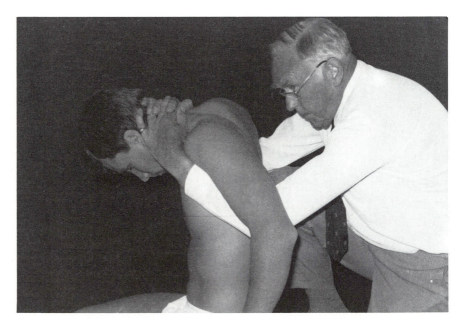

Fig. 8.14 Alternative sitting high velocity treatment for thoracic spine for ERS$_R$; position before thrust.

(d) Introduce your right hand through her right axilla and grip her right wrist. While adjusting her position, you use your left hand to monitor tension at T6–7.

(e) Place your left foot on a support of such a height that it will allow you to rest the front of your left knee against the back of the left transverse process of T7. With your right hand, introduce flexion by translating T6–7 backwards. Do not block this movement with your knee.

(f) With your right hand, rotate her upper trunk to the left and sidebend her to the left at the same time. This and the previous movement must be controlled so that the tension is brought to the T6 level.

(g) Maintain the patient's position but insert your left hand through her left axilla and grip her left wrist.

(h) Ask her to exhale to help flexion and give a sharp pull with both hands in a direction that is more superior than posterior. This will flex and rotate T6 to the left with some sidebending.

Technique 8c

Sitting technique for neutral dysfunction of the lower thoracic spine with restriction of left rotation and right sidebending at T5–6–7–8 (N_R) (see Fig. 8.13).

1. Diagnostic points.

(a) With the patient erect, T5, 6 and 7 are rotated to the right (right transverse processes posterior).

(b) With the patient either flexed or extended, a right rotation of the three vertebrae remains although it may alter in degree.

2. Treatment.

(a) The patient sits on a stool or with her legs over the side of the table.

(b) You stand behind her and you may need a stool with cross bars or some other support that will enable you to rest your foot at the required height. (Sometimes it is possible to use the table itself.)

(c) Ask her to lace her fingers behind the base of her neck with her elbows forward.

(d) Introduce your right hand through her right axilla and grip her right wrist. While adjusting her position, use your left hand to monitor tension at T6–7.

(e) Place your left foot on a support of such a height that it will allow you to rest the front of your left knee against the back of the left transverse process of T7. Do not introduce either flexion or extension.

(f) With your right hand, rotate her upper trunk to the left and sidebend her to the right at the same time. This must be controlled so that the tension is brought to the T6 level.

(g) Maintain the patient's position but insert your left hand through her left axilla and grip her left wrist.

(h) Give a sharp pull superiorly and posteriorly with both hands. This will rotate T6 to the left with right sidebending.

THE UPPER THORACIC SPINE

For this region also, a wide variety of techniques has been described.

Sitting techniques

These can use either muscle energy or high velocity activating force. As in the sitting techniques for the lower thoracic spine, reliance is placed on the weight of the patient to stabilise the bones below the level of the dysfunction.

Technique 9a

For extension restriction. Described for T3 with restriction of rotation and sidebending to the left (FRS$_R$) (Fig. 8.15).

1. Diagnostic points.
(a) With the patient erect, the right transverse process of T3 may be slightly more prominent (posterior) than the left.
(b) When the patient flexes, the transverse processes of T3 are nearly or completely level; the right transverse process goes forward to be level with the left.

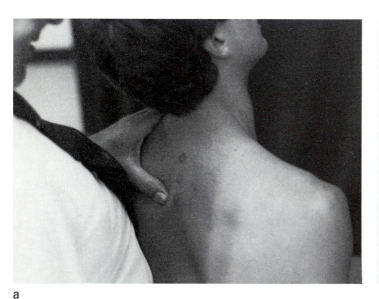
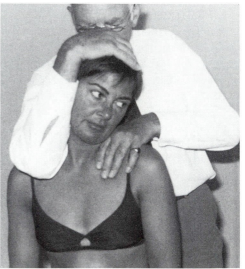

a   b

Fig. 8.15 Sitting treatment for upper thoracic spine FRS$_R$: **(a)** position of your left hand, **(b)** the position before the effort (or thrust).

(c) When the patient extends, the right transverse process of T3 becomes more posterior, the left transverse process does not come down and back.

2. Treatment.

(a) The patient sits on a stool or with her legs over the side of the table. It is important that she should 'sit up tall'.

(b) You stand behind her.

(c) Place your left hand over the 'shawl' area of her left shoulder and contact the back of the left transverse process of T3 with your thumb.

(d) Lean forward enough to support her trunk with your chest.

(e) Place your right arm or elbow on the top of her right shoulder and rest your hand on her head, holding her neck in slight left sidebending. The position of your right arm should be adjusted by sliding the elbow forwards or backwards so that your forearm is close to the side of the patient's neck, and the force to be exerted by the sidebending of her head will be transmitted by your forearm to her shoulder, thus protecting her cervical spine. The precise position will depend on the relative lengths of your forearm and her neck.

(f) Tell the patient to allow you to arch her back, which you do by pressure from your left thumb and slight extension of her neck. This position must be controlled to bring the tension to the level of your thumb. This will translate T3 forward at the apex of the curve.

(g) Use the web of your left hand to translate T3 to the right in order to produce a left sidebend with apex at T3. This movement also is monitored by your left thumb.

(h) With your right hand, rotate her head to the left until you feel the accumulation of tension at the T3 level. You have now reached the barrier in all three planes.

(i) Muscle energy variant.

    (i) Ask her to attempt to push her head to the right (or ask her to attempt to flex her upper back) while you resist with an equal and opposite force.

    (ii) After 4 or 5 seconds both relax, but do not lose the position.

    (iii) After full relaxation, take up the slack by further extension and sidebending.

    (iv) Repeat steps (i), (ii) and (iii) three or four times.

(j) High velocity variant.

    (i) Move your left thumb against the left side of the spinous process of T3.

    (ii) With the web of your hand on her trapezius and the tip of your thumb against the spinous process of T3, give a short sharp thrust downwards and to the right to produce left sidebending and left rotation in extension. At the same time, slightly increase the pressure to the left on her head with your right hand.

(k) Retest.

Technique 9b

For flexion restriction. Described for T3 with restriction of rotation and sidebending to the left (ERS$_R$) (Fig. 8.16).

1. Diagnostic points.
(a) With the patient erect, the right transverse process of T3 may be slightly more prominent (posterior) than the left.
(b) When the patient flexes the neck, the right transverse process of T3 does not go forward and the left becomes relatively higher and less prominent.
(c) When the patient extends the neck, the left transverse process comes down and back to be level with the right.
2. Treatment.
(a) The patient sits on a stool or with her legs over the side of the table. It is important that she should 'sit up tall'.
(b) You stand behind her.
(c) Place your left hand over the 'shawl' area of her left shoulder and contact the back of the left transverse process of T3 with your thumb.
(d) Lean forward enough to support her trunk with your chest.
(e) Place your right arm or elbow on the top of her right shoulder and rest your hand on her head, holding her neck in slight left sidebending. (See technique 9a para. 2(e).)
(f) Ask her to 'slump' against your chest just far enough to bring the

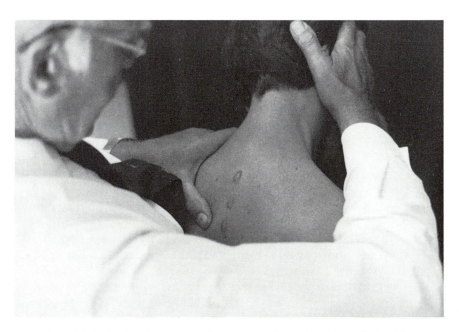

Fig. 8.16 Sitting treatment for upper thoracic spine ERS$_R$. The positioning of the operator's right hand and arm has not been completed to allow the remainder to be seen; it should end up as in Fig. 8.15(b).

tension to the level of your thumb and translate T3 backwards to form the apex of the curve.

(g) Use the web of your left hand to translate T3 to the right in order to produce a left sidebend with apex at T3. This movement also is monitored by your left thumb.

(h) With your right hand rotate her head to the left until you feel the accumulation of tension at the T3 level. You have now reached the barrier in all three planes.

(i) Muscle energy variant.

    (i) Ask her to attempt to push her head to the right (or ask her to attempt to extend her upper back) while you resist with an equal and opposite force.

    (ii) After 4 or 5 seconds both relax, but do not lose the position.

    (iii) After full relaxation, take up the slack by further flexion and sidebending.

    (iv) Repeat steps (i), (ii) and (iii) three or four times.

(j) High velocity variant.

    (i) Move your left thumb against the left side of the spinous process of T3.

    (ii) With the web of your hand on her trapezius and the tip of your thumb against the spinous process of T3, give a short sharp thrust downwards and to the right to produce left sidebending and left rotation in flexion. At the same time, slightly increase the pressure to the left on her head with your right hand.

(k) Retest.

Technique 9c

For neutral dysfunction. Described for T2–3–4–5 with restriction of rotation to the right and sidebending to the left (N_L) (Fig. 8.17).

1. Diagnostic points.

(a) With the patient erect, T2, 3 and 4 are rotated to the left (left transverse processes posterior).

(b) With the patient either flexed or extended, a left rotation of the three vertebrae remains although it may alter in degree.

2. Treatment.

(a) The patient sits on a stool or with her legs over the side of the table. It is important that she should 'sit up tall'.

(b) You stand behind her.

(c) Place your left hand over the 'shawl' area of her left shoulder and contact the back of the left transverse process of T3 with your thumb.

(d) Lean forward enough to support her trunk with your chest.

(e) Place your right arm or elbow on the top of her right shoulder and rest your hand on her head, holding her neck in slight left sidebending. (See technique 9a para. 2(e).)

(f) Do not allow her to slump or to hyperextend.

(g) Use the web of your left hand to translate T3 to the right in order

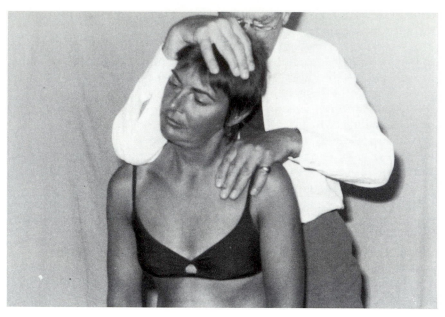

Fig. 8.17 Sitting treatment for upper thoracic spine N_L. Note the different rotation of the head.

to produce a left sidebend with apex at T3. This movement also is monitored by your left thumb.

(h) With your right hand, rotate her head to the right until you feel the accumulation of tension at the T3 level. You have now reached the barrier.

(i) Muscle energy variant.

(i) Ask her to attempt to push her head to the right while you resist with an equal and opposite force.

(ii) After 4 or 5 seconds both relax, but do not lose the position.

(iii) After full relaxation, take up the slack by further flexion and sidebending.

(iv) Repeat steps (i),(ii) and (iii) three or four times.

(j) High velocity variant.

(i) Press forwards with your left thumb against the left transverse process of T3 until you reach the rotation barrier.

(ii) With the web of your hand on her trapezius, give a short sharp thrust downwards and to the right to produce left sidebending, and increase the pressure forwards with your thumb to produce right rotation. At the same time, slightly increase the pressure to the left on her head with your right hand.

(k) Retest.

Supine techniques

These use high velocity thrusting. They are very similar to technique 5 but the arms are placed in a different manner to control the upper vertebrae better. This difference means that some of the pressure applied is transmitted through the ribs and care must be taken to avoid too great a force.

The variant using one arm only across the chest has been associated with costochondral junction injury and is best avoided. These techniques should not be used if there is much soreness in the anterior chest wall.

They are hybrid techniques using a short lever (the transverse process) below and a long lever above. Accurate localisation from above is essential; the contact below is on the vertebra itself and localisation is automatic.

Technique 10a

For restriction of flexion. Supine treatment of type II upper thoracic dysfunction, described for restriction of left rotation and sidebending at T3–4 (ERS$_R$) (Fig. 8.18).

A modification of this technique can be used to treat external torsion of the corresponding rib at the same time. This is described in Chapter 11.

1. Diagnostic points.
(a) With the patient erect, the right transverse process of T3 may be slightly more prominent (posterior) than the left.
(b) When the patient flexes the neck, the right transverse process of T3 does not go forward and the left becomes relatively higher and less prominent.
(c) When the patient extends the neck, the left transverse process comes down and back to be level with the right.

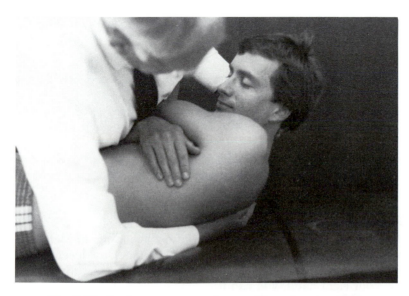

Fig. 8.18 Supine treatment of upper thoracic spine, ERS$_R$.

2. Treatment.

The patient lies on her back.

(f) You stand on her right (the side to which T3 is rotated).

(g) Ask her to cross her arms over her chest, left on top, so that the fingers are in the axillae. The right arm should be on top when you are treating a left rotated vertebra.

(h) Lift her left shoulder with your left hand until you can get your right hand under her at the level to be treated. Your right hand should be held so that it can support the transverse processes on either side at the vertebra below the joint to be treated. This is best accomplished by flexing the interphalangeal joints but leaving the meta-carpophalangeal joints extended. The patient's spinous processes are then cradled in the groove, and the base of your thenar eminence should support the left transverse process of T4.

(e) Allow her shoulder to return to the table top with your hand under her.

(f) Slide your left hand down under the patient's head until your fingertips reach her upper thorax. Then lift her head and neck until the tension reaches your right thumb at the T3 level.

(g) Use your left hand and forearm to rotate and sidebend her head to the left until you feel the tension reach T3 (with your right thumb).

(h) When the barrier has been engaged in all three planes, lean over so that you can press down on her elbows with your chest. The elbows can be padded with a small pillow if desired. The thrust is then given by a short sharp increase in the pressure with your body in the direction of the base of your right thenar eminence.

(i) Retest.

Technique 10b

For restriction of extension. Described for restriction of left rotation and sidebending at T3–4 (FRS$_R$) (Fig. 8.19).

1. Diagnostic points.

(a) With the patient erect, the right transverse process of T3 may be slightly more prominent (posterior) than the left.

(b) When the patient flexes, the transverse processes of T3 are nearly or completely level, the right transverse process goes forward to be level with the left.

(c) When the patient extends, the right transverse process of T3 becomes more posterior, the left transverse process does not come down and back.

2. Treatment.

Steps (a) to (e) are as for the flexion restricted lesion.

(f) With your left hand, introduce left sidebending and left rotation of her head and neck until you feel the tension reach the level of T3.

(g) By contracting the muscles of your right thenar eminence, or by lifting your right hand, you can fine tune the extension position so that the barrier is engaged in all three planes.

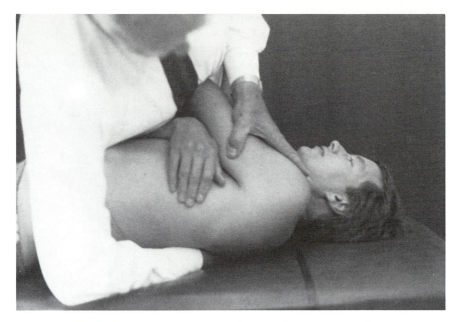

Fig. 8.19 Supine treatment of upper thoracic spine, FRS$_R$.

(h) The thrust is given as before in the direction of the base of your right thenar eminence.

Technique 10c

For neutral dysfunction. Described for restriction of right sidebending and of left rotation at T2–3–4–5 (N$_R$) (Fig. 8.20).

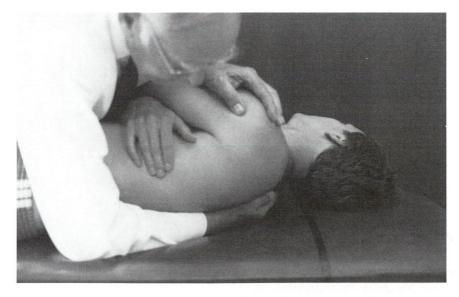

Fig. 8.20 Supine treatment of upper thoracic spine, N$_R$.

1. Diagnostic points.

(a) With the patient erect, T2, 3 and 4 are rotated to the right (right transverse processes posterior).

(b) With the patient either flexed or extended, a right rotation of the three vertebrae remains although it may alter in degree.

2. Treatment.

Steps (a) to (e) as in the treatment for flexion restriction.

(f) With your left hand, lift her left shoulder enough to restore neutral flexion/extension to her thoracic spine.

(g) Use your left hand and forearm to rotate her upper trunk to the left and sidebend it to the right; in each case the movement must be monitored and stopped when the tension just reaches T3.

(h) The thrust is given as before in the direction of the base of your right thenar eminence.

Prone techniques

These are the specific variants of the *chin pivot thrust* described in Chapter 9. There is no good specific variant of this technique for restrictions of flexion.

Technique 11a

Prone high velocity treatment for restricted extension. Described for restriction of left rotation and sidebending at T2-3 (FRS$_R$) (Fig. 8.21).

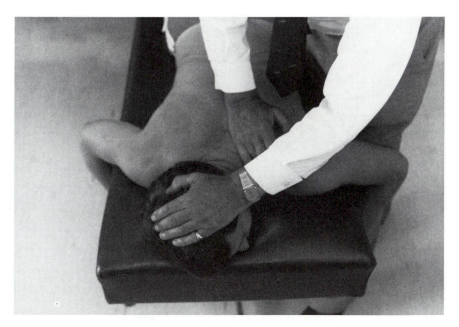

Fig. 8.21 Prone high velocity treatment for upper thoracic spine, FRS$_R$.

1. Diagnostic points.

(a) With the patient erect, the right transverse process of T2 may be slightly more prominent (posterior) than the left.

(b) When the patient flexes, the transverse processes of T2 are nearly or completely level, the right transverse process goes forward to be level with the left.

(c) When the patient extends, the right transverse process of T2 becomes more posterior, the left transverse process does not come down and back.

2. Treatment.

(a) The patient lies prone. Any hole or slot in the table is better closed.

(b) You stand to her left near the head of the table.

(c) Monitor for tension with your right hand at the T2 level.

(d) Raise her head slightly and extend the neck, then rotate and sidebend it to the left until the tension reaches your right hand.

(e) Rest her head on the right side of her chin and control rotation with your left hand on the back of her head.

(f) Bring your right pisiform up to the caudal aspect of the left transverse process of T3.

(g) Thrust with your right hand craniad and anteriorly while you slightly increase the pressure with your left hand.

(h) Retest.

Technique 11b

For neutral dysfunction. Described for restriction of right sidebending and left rotation at T2–3 (N_R) (Fig. 8.22).

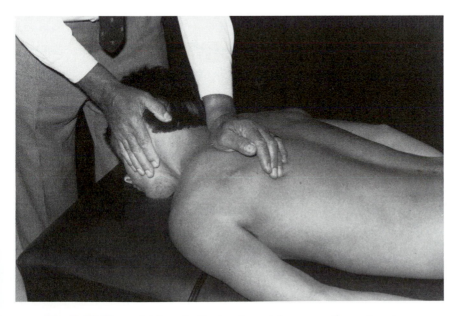

Fig. 8.22 Prone high velocity treatment for upper thoracic spine, N_R.

1. Diagnostic points.

(a) With the patient erect, T1, 2 and 3 are rotated to the left (left transverse processes posterior).

(b) With the patient either flexed or extended, a left rotation of the three vertebrae remains although it may alter in degree.

2. Treatment.

(a) The patient lies prone.

(b) You stand at the head of the table.

(c) Monitor with your left hand at the T2 level.

(d) With your right hand, lift her head into extension and sidebend her neck a little to the right. Allow her to rest on her chin.

(e) Introduce left rotation and increase the right sidebending by pivoting her head to the right on her chin until you feel the tension just reach T2. If it seems to need too much rotation to reach the barrier, more sidebending should first be introduced by moving her chin to the right on the table top.

(f) Contact the posterosuperior aspect of the left transverse process of T3 with your left pisiform.

(g) Give a short sharp thrust anteriorly and caudad on the left transverse process of T3 while slightly increasing your pressure to the right on her head.

Chapter 9

Treatment of the Lumbar and Thoracic Spine, Semispecific

PRINCIPLES

The basic principles are the same as those outlined in Chapter 8. Here, the application is different.

The diagnostic point of first importance is the level of the dysfunction to be treated. In this approach it is determined by the absence or restriction of motion at an individual level and by the presence on one side of significant soft tissue tension.

The direction of thrust is deduced from the location of the tissue tension abnormality.

This is a simpler approach than the fully specific and it seems that it would be unlikely to do enough good. The experience of one of the authors, however, is that very often it does what is required. He used this approach for many years before he learnt any better and the results were good, although it is probable that they would have been better if the fully specific approach had been used.

As previously stated, it is the authors' belief that semispecific localisation is not good enough if muscle energy is to be used as the activating force. The treatments to be described will all use high velocity, low amplitude thrusting.

In patients with very acute lesions where there is widespread muscle spasm, it is difficult to make a confident diagnosis by this method. It is unwise to perform a high velocity treatment in such cases except for those with experience.

THE LUMBAR SPINE

Technique A

Described for restriction of motion at L4–5, with the maximum soft tissue tension on the left side (see Figs. 9.1, 9.2, 9.3). If the maximum soft tissue tension had been on the right, the description would be the same but with the sides reversed. The movement used in this technique is rotation and it is important to remember that the range of rotation in the lumbar spine is very small.

1. The patient lies on her right side.
2. You stand facing her.
3. Monitor at the L4–5 level with your free hand.
4. With your right hand, bend up her left hip and knee to the point when you feel the tissue tension just reach L5. The final adjustment can often be made more easily if you control her leg with your abdomen. This allows you to monitor with both hands. Make sure that you have not 'locked' L4–5 by too much flexion.
5. Without changing the flexion/extension position, put down her left leg so that the foot hangs over the edge of the table. If it seems likely that she will attempt to move her leg, you can hold its position by putting your right leg over it to prevent extension of the hip.
6. Pull her right shoulder forward to rotate her trunk to the left until you feel the tension begin to rise at the L3–4 level, note that this is one above that to be treated.
7. The spine is now 'locked' from above by rotation and a slight sidebend and from below by flexion (Fig. 9.1a, b and c).
8. Long lever variant.
(a) Put your left arm through her left axilla and place your fingers

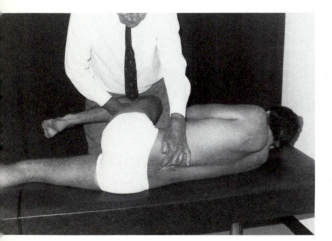
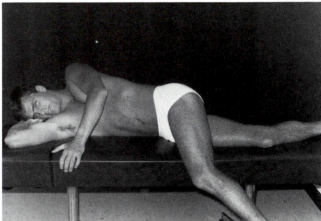
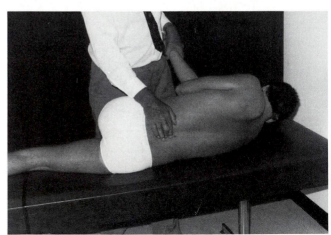

Fig. 9.1 'Locking' the lumbar spine: **(a)** from below, **(b)** position after locking from below, **(c)** from above.

so that they can monitor tension at the L3–4–5 levels. The position described for the left arm in the hybrid variant can be used instead.

(b) Use your right fingers also as monitors at the lesion and place your forearm so that you can press on her left buttock halfway between the ASIS and the ischial tuberosity.

(c) Ask her to take three deep breaths in and out and each time take up the slack by increasing the rotation, but only up to the barrier.

(d) The treatment is given by a short sharp thrust forwards on her left buttock and backwards on her left shoulder. The main force is applied to the buttock (Fig. 9.2a and b). It is vital that the patient should be relaxed. If she is not, the force required to perform a movement will be greater than it is advisable to use.

9. Hybrid variant. This uses a short lever on the caudal side and positioning from below is less critical, although it still helps the movement.

(a) Lean over the patient and, with your wrist extended, contact the posterior aspect of the left transverse process of her L5 with your right

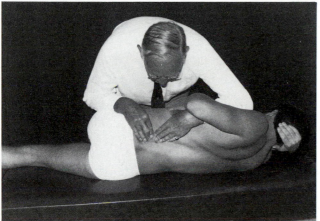

a

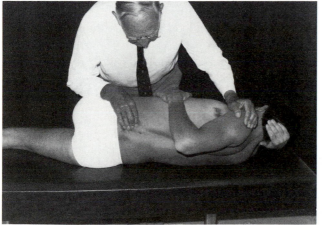

b

Fig. 9.2 Position for long lever thrust: **(a)** using both hands to monitor, **(b)** using one hand to monitor.

pisiform bone. Your forearm should be horizontal and extending backwards perpendicular to her trunk.

(b) Press back gently on her left shoulder with your left hand to take up the slack. (It is not possible to get your left hand into position to monitor and that must be done by your right hand, although its position is not ideal.)

(c) Ask her to take three deep breaths in and out and each time take up the slack by increasing the rotation, but only up to the barrier.

(d) The treatment is given by a very short sharp thrust forwards (towards you) by your right pisiform while you somewhat increase the counterpressure with your left hand (Fig. 9.3).

10. Retest.

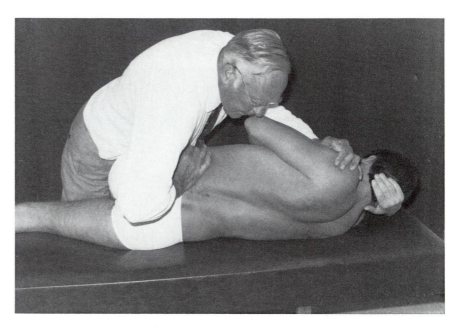

Fig. 9.3 Position for thrust in hybrid variant.

THE LOWER THORACIC SPINE

The lowest joints are often best treated by lumbar techniques, but these become increasingly difficult above T11. The supine treatment for the mid thoracic levels is difficult in some patients below about T10, but the crossed pisiform technique can be used even as low as the upper lumbar joints if necessary.

Patients with an unusually wide range of motion in their joints can be difficult to treat. This applies particularly to the supine techniques and in some cases a different method must be used. The difficulty is chiefly one of localisation of force, the range of motion may be so wide that it is impossible to bring the tension down to the required level in the supine position.

When using this approach it is often easiest to have the patient supine when assessing the location of the tissue tension abnormality. For the lowest joints, the prone position or that used for the lumbar spine may be easier. For the uppermost joints, the sitting position is usually the easiest. All of these are described in Chapter 5.

Technique B

Supine. Described for restriction of motion at T6–7, with maximum tissue tension on the left side (Fig. 9.4). This is the semispecific variant of specific technique 6 described in Chapter 8. It is a hybrid technique

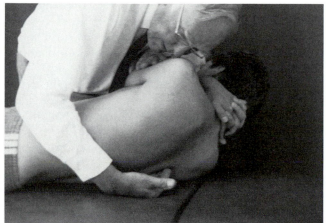

a

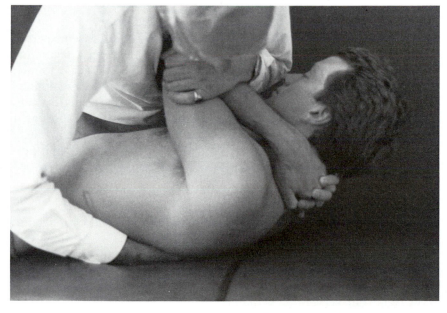

b

Fig. 9.4 Supine treatment for stiffness at T6–7 with hypertonus on the left: (a) to show hand placement, (b) position for thrust.

using a long lever above and a short lever below and produces a gapping of the joint in flexion, with some right rotation of T6.

1. The patient lies on her back.
2. You stand facing her right side.
3. Ask her to lace her fingers together behind the base of her neck. It is important that the hands are as low as possible to avoid uncomfortable hyperflexion of the neck.
4. Lift her left shoulder with your left hand and roll her upper trunk towards you until you can get your right hand behind her at the level of the joint to be treated. Your right hand should be partly flexed at the metacarpophalangeal joints to provide a trough for the spinous processes. The base of your thenar eminence (the tubercle of the scaphoid) should be in contact with the left transverse process of her T7. Your fingers support the right side of her spine and may be flexed at the interphalangeal joints to provide more support. Your right thumb points craniad and serves to monitor the tissue tension.
5. Roll her back to the supine position with your right hand underneath.
6. With your left hand, flex her trunk by pulling caudad on her elbows until you feel the tension just reach the T5–6 level.
7. Lean over her so that your chest can press on her elbows (and your left hand).
8. Thrust at the end of exhalation by a sudden increase in the pressure with your chest in the direction of your right carpal scaphoid.
9. Retest.

Technique C

Prone, for thoracic spine (T4 to L1) (Fig. 9.5). This is a semispecific version of the *crossed pisiform* technique described as specific technique 7. It is particularly useful for restrictions of extension but is easy to misuse and the previous warning is repeated here. It is a short lever technique and, although this makes localisation automatic, it means that great care must be taken to ensure that the force is stopped almost as soon as it starts. 'The movement at the joint is less than an eighth of an inch' (3 mm). Attention to the detail of the technique is important as, if performed carelessly, the costovertebral joints can be damaged. Described for restriction of motion at T6–7, with the maximum tissue tension on the right.

1. The patient lies prone, preferably with her nose and chin accommodated by a slot in the table.
2. You stand on the side of the maximum tissue tension (the right side in this example).
3. Bring your left pisiform bone into contact with the caudal aspect of the right transverse process of her T6.
4. Cross your hands to bring your right pisiform against the posterior surface of the left transverse process of T7.
5. Ask her to inhale, to produce some extension of the spine.

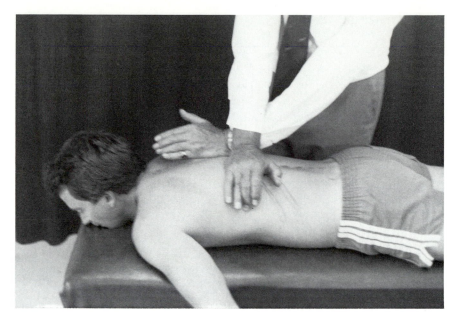

Fig. 9.5 Prone treatment for stiffness at T6–7 with hypertonus on the right.

6. Give a *very short* sharp thrust with both hands simultaneously. The direction of the thrust is important. With your right hand, it should be anterior and slightly craniad; with your left hand, it should be craniad and only slightly anterior.

7. As always, retest.

Technique D

Sitting for the thoracic spine (T4 to about T10). Described for stiffness at T6–7, with maximum tension on the right (Fig. 9.6). This technique

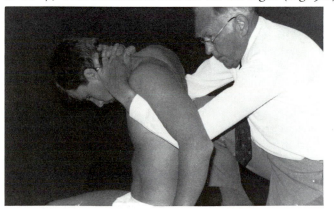
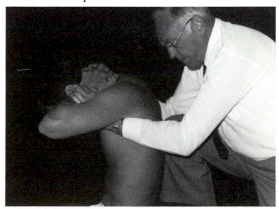

a

b

Fig. 9.6 Sitting treatment for thoracic spine: **(a)** with your fingers laced behind the patient's neck, **(b)** with you gripping the patient's wrists.

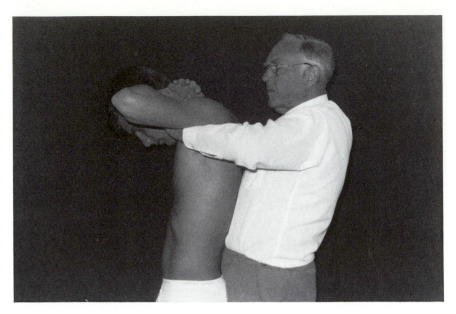

Fig. 9.7 Using the abdomen as fulcrum in treating the thoracic spine, shown standing.

has a number of variants and can be made fully specific or at least very nearly so. It can also be done standing, using one's lower chest as a fulcrum and, although in that form its effect is more that of a general distraction, it can at times be surprisingly helpful. That is one of the very few ways in which it may be possible to help someone in circumstances which preclude examination.

1. The patient sits on a stool or with her legs over the side of the table.

2. You stand behind her.

3. Put your arms through her axillae and *either* lace your fingers behind the base of her neck (Fig. 9.6a) . . .

4. *or* have her lace her fingers behind the base of her neck and you take hold of her wrists (Fig. 9.6b).

5. Place a fulcrum against her back. It is often most easily done by using one of your knees. If the knee is bony, it is kind to put a pad between it and her spine. Your lower chest or abdomen is less specific but sometimes easier to use, and the manipulation can then be performed with patient and operator standing (Fig. 9.7). A pad can also be used here, especially for those who are thin.

6. The correct positioning of the fulcrum determines the specificity. If the knee is used, it is necessary to have the foot supported at a level that will allow you to have your knee at the right height. A stool with a series of horizontal bars is very useful for the purpose. Clearly, the shape of the abdomen makes it much more difficult to adjust the level of that fulcrum accurately. A small firm cushion can help in this respect. The fulcrum should be placed so that its pressure is applied to the vertebra below the joint to be treated. The optimum place is such that

the pressure comes on the back of the transverse process of (in this example) T7 on the side to which T7 is relatively rotated. This will often be the side of the maximum tissue tension at the T6–7 level and, for the semispecific application, that is the side to choose.

7. Adjust the flexion/extension position to that which gives the best concentration of tension at the T6–7 level. It will be easier for some operators to use one hand to monitor this before taking up the full position. The patient can be controlled with only one arm in position (see the description of technique 8 in Chapter 8). If the restriction is mainly of flexion, the position adopted should be in flexion. If the restriction is extension, the position can be adjusted by altering the line of pull of the arms.

8. The treatment is given by a short sharp pull upward and backward with your arms and is best done at the end of exhalation. If the pull is more upward, the joint will be flexed; if more backward, it will be extended.

9. Retest.

THE UPPER THORACIC SPINE

A prone and a supine technique will be described. The prone method is better when there is restriction of extension, the supine for a restriction of flexion.

Technique E

Supine treatment for upper thoracic dysfunction. Described for stiffness at T2–3, with maximum tissue tension on the left side (Fig. 9.8). This is the semispecific variant of technique 10 described in Chapter 8. It is very similar to technique B but the arms are placed in a different manner to control the upper vertebrae better. This difference means that some of the pressure applied is transmitted through the ribs and care must be taken to avoid too great a force. The technique should not be used if there is much soreness in the front of the upper ribs. The variant using only one arm across the chest has been associated with costochondral joint injury and is best avoided.

1. The patient lies on her back.
2. You stand on her right.
3. Cross her arms over her chest with the elbows in the midline and the right arm next to the chest wall.
4. With your left hand, lift her left shoulder and roll her towards you enough to get your right hand under her at the T3 level.
5. Your hand placement is the same (except for level) as in technique B. The base of your right thenar eminence (the tubercle of the scaphoid) supports the left transverse process of her T3. Your fingers support the other side of her spine and your right thumb points cranially beside the spinous processes where it serves as monitor.

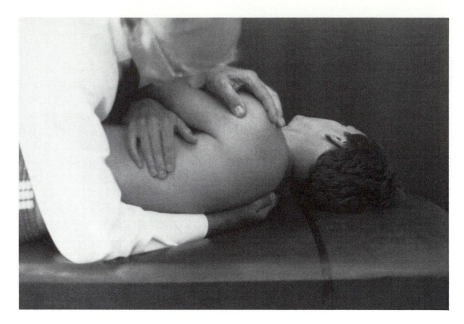

Fig. 9.8 Supine treatment for upper thoracic spine
with hypertonus on the left.

6. Roll her back onto your hand.

7. With your left hand, pull caudally and to the right on her left
shoulder until you feel the tension reach T2. This introduces flexion
and right rotation.

8. Treat by a short sharp thrust given with the front of your chest
leaning over her crossed elbows. The thrust should be directed towards
your right carpal scaphoid.

9. Retest.

Technique F

Prone technique for the upper thoracic spine (Fig. 9.9). This is a semispecific variant of the chin pivot thrust technique described in Chapter 8.
It is a very powerful technique and has the advantage that it is more
difficult for even a tense patient to resist than most other methods. It
is primarily for those with restriction of extension, but if the rotation
is corrected, it will often be found to be effective even in those where
the sagittal plane restriction is of flexion. Described for stiffness at T2–3,
with maximum tissue tension on the left side.

1. The patient lies prone. Any hole or slot for the nose and chin should
be closed or the patient moved away from it.

2. You stand facing the head of the table.

3. With your right hand, lift her head, extend the neck and let her
rest on her chin.

4. With your left pisiform, contact the posterosuperior aspect of the
left transverse process of her T3.

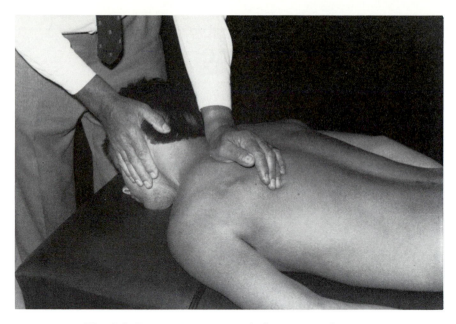

Fig. 9.9 Prone treatment of the upper thoracic spine with hypertonus on the left.

5. While monitoring with your left hand, use your right to pivot her head on her chin to the right. This introduces right sidebending and left rotation and must be stopped when the tension reaches T2.

6. Ask her to breathe deeply and, at the end of exhalation, give a short sharp thrust anteriorly and slightly caudad on the transverse process of T3 while you simultaneously increase the right sidebending of the head.

7. Retest.

Cervicothoracic junction: even the last two techniques may be difficult in this area and the techniques described for the lower cervical levels can be useful here.

Chapter 10

Treatment of the Cervical Spine

WARNING

In previous editions of this book, descriptions were given of high velocity treatment for all of the joints of the cervical spine. The First Edition was written before muscle energy treatment was first described and at that time high velocity, low amplitude thrusting was the standard form of manipulation for all regions of the spine.

As is now well known, there have been a number of accidents in which more or less serious results have been recorded, even involving the death of the patient. The problem has been one of damage to (or sometimes only spasm in) arteries in the vertebrobasilar axis, and in the more serious cases there has been thrombosis with permanent sequelae. Accidents may be more likely in those with atherosclerosis but they have happened in young healthy patients also.

It appears that all the accidents have been due to a high velocity manipulation, or to positioning in extreme extension prior to such manipulation, or, very infrequently, to a pre-existing vascular abnormality (such as a dissecting aneurysm).

The authors no longer feel justified in including high velocity techniques for the occipitoatlantal or atlantoaxial joints and these will not be found in this edition. Fortunately, muscle energy treatment for these joints is effective and not difficult to learn, nor is the fully specific diagnosis difficult at these levels.

Specific and semispecific treatment will be described for the 'typical' cervical joints.

It is worth noting that all the supine techniques described follow naturally from the position required for the supine examination of the same joint. In a similar manner, the sitting techniques follow from the position necessary for the dynamic assessment of motion in the cervicothoracic area described in Chapter 5.

THE OCCIPITOATLANTAL JOINT

At this joint there is a small amount of rotation which is coupled to sidebending according to type I spinal movement. The range is so small that no special care need to be taken to introduce that movement.

Sometimes it will be found that there is restriction in both flexion and extension. In that case both should be treated.

Technique 1

For restricted flexion, described for restriction of right sidebending (Fig. 10.1).

1. Diagnostic points.

(a) With the chin tipped down, the head will not translate fully to the left.

(b) With the chin tipped up, translation to the sides is equal.

(c) There is no major restriction of sidebending in the lower cervical joints.

2. Treatment.

(a) The patient is supine.

(b) You stand or sit at the head of the table.

(c) Cradle her head in your hands in such a way that you can monitor for movement of C1 with your index or middle fingers. Your monitoring fingers should be lateral and not over the occipitoatlantal membrane.

(d) Tilt her head gently so that it is slightly chin down.

(e) Sidebend her head on the neck to the right at the occipitoatlantal joint until you feel the tension begin to rise. If C1 moves, you have gone too far.

(f) Ask her to attempt to sidebend her head gently to the left while you resist the movement. Gentle force is all that is required, you are working with small muscles.

(g) After 4 or 5 seconds both relax, but do not lose the position.

(h) When she has relaxed fully (and not before), take up the slack by further sidebending to the new barrier.

(i) Repeat steps (f), (g) and (h) three or four times.

(j) Retest.

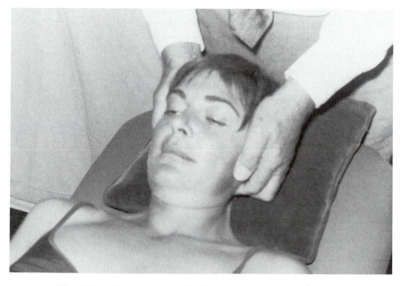

Fig. 10.1 Treatment of the occipitoatlantal joint with restricted flexion.

Technique 2

For restricted extension, described for restriction of right sidebending (Fig. 10.2).

1. Diagnostic points.

(a) With the chin tipped up, the head will not translate fully to the left.

(b) With the chin tipped down, translation to the sides is equal.

(c) There is no major restriction of sidebending in the lower cervical joints.

2. Treatment.

(a) The patient is supine.

(b) You stand or sit at the head of the table.

(c) Cradle her head in your hands in such a way that you can monitor for movement of C1 with your index or middle fingers. Your monitoring fingers should be lateral and not over the occipitoatlantal membrane.

(d) Tilt her head gently so that it is slightly chin up. *Do not extend the neck or fully extend the head on the neck.*

(e) Sidebend her head on the neck to the right at the occipitoatlantal joint until you feel the tension begin to rise. If C1 moves, you have gone too far.

(f) Ask her to attempt to sidebend her head gently to the left while you resist the movement. Gentle force is all that is required, you are working with small muscles.

(g) After 4 or 5 seconds both relax, but do not lose the position.

(h) When she has relaxed fully (and not before), take up the slack by further sidebending to the new barrier.

(i) Repeat steps (f), (g) and (h) three or four times.

(j) Retest.

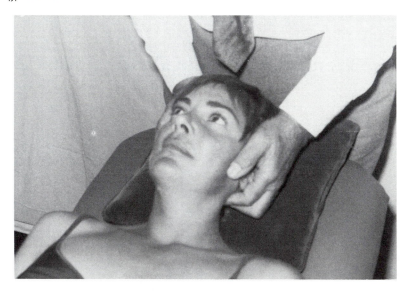

Fig. 10.2 Treatment of the occipitoatlantal joint with restricted extension.

THE ATLANTOAXIAL JOINT

Technique 3

There is more rotation at this joint than at any other in the cervical spine. It is therefore of some clinical interest that even in patients with marked loss of rotation in the neck, the rotatory range at this joint may be nearly or completely normal when tested as outlined in Chapter 5.

1. Diagnostic point.
(a) With the neck flexed as far as it easily goes, there is restriction of rotation of the head to one side.
2. Treatment, described for restriction of rotation to the left (Fig. 10.3).
(a) The patient lies supine.
(b) You stand or sit at her head.
(c) Lift her head in both your hands and monitor with your fingers laterally at the C1–2 level.
(d) Flex the neck to the point when you feel the sense of barrier with your monitoring fingers. This will usually be near the limit of easy motion.
(e) Rotate the head and atlas to the left until you feel the tension begin to rise at the C1 level.
(f) Hold the head with your left hand while you move your right hand to the right side of her face.
(g) Ask her to attempt gently to rotate her head to the right against your resistance. It is important to emphasise the small force required, nearly all patients will try too hard.

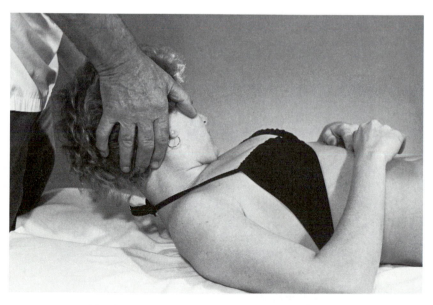

Fig. 10.3 Treatment of the atlantoaxial joint.

(h) After 4 or 5 seconds both relax.

(i) When she has relaxed fully (and not before), take up the slack to the new barrier by rotation.

(j) Repeat steps (g), (h) and (i) three or four times.

(k) Retest.

THE TYPICAL CERVICAL JOINTS, C2 TO T1

The joints from C2 down to T1 always move in the type II mode and there is no neutral dysfunction to be treated at these levels.

Technique 4

Supine treatment for restriction of extension. Described for restriction of sidebending and rotation to the left at C4–5 (FRS$_R$) (Fig. 10.4).

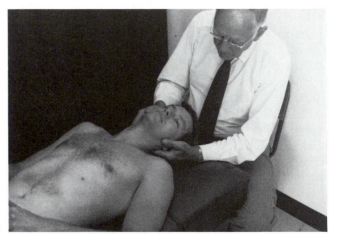

a

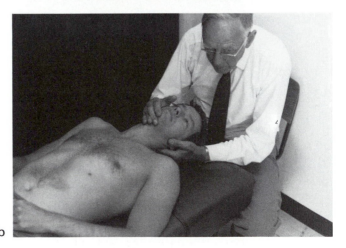

b

Fig. 10.4 Treatment of typical cervical joints (C2–7) for FRS$_R$: **(a)** using sidebend effort, **(b)** using flexion effort.

1. Diagnostic points.

(a) On translation to the right at the C4 level, there is restriction of movement usually associated with tenderness. Translation to the left is free.

(b) The restriction is worse when the neck is extended and usually disappears when it is flexed.

2. Treatment.

(a) The patient lies supine.

(b) You stand or sit at her head.

(c) With your left index or middle finger, contact the back of the left articular pillar of C5. For this dysfunction, your monitoring finger should be at the lower vertebra to encourage extension.

(d) Lift anteriorly until you feel the tension just reach your fingertip. That point is usually tender and it may help if you ask her to allow you to arch her neck; she must not do it herself because that will not be likely to stop at the required point. For this step some prefer to use the finger of the other hand on the right side as well.

(e) With your right hand on the right side of her head, introduce sidebending and rotation to the left until you feel the tension reach the C4 level.

(f) Ask the patient to make a gentle effort to sidebend to the right *or* to attempt to nod her head gently. If flexion is to be the effort, the fingers of your right hand should support her under the chin so that you can resist the effort. Rotation could be used but is more difficult for the operator to control.

(g) After 4 or 5 seconds both relax, but do not the lose the position.

(h) When she has relaxed fully (and not before), take up the slack by extension and sidebending to the new barrier.

(i) Repeat steps (f), (g) and (h) three or four times.

(j) Retest.

Technique 5

Supine treatment for restriction of flexion. Described for restriction of sidebending and rotation to the left at C4–5 (ERS$_R$) (Fig. 10.5).

1. Diagnostic points.

(a) On translation to the right at the C4 level, there is restriction of movement usually associated with tenderness. Translation to the left is free.

(b) The restriction is worse when the neck is flexed and usually disappears when it is extended.

2. Treatment.

(a) The patient lies supine.

(b) You stand or sit at her head.

(c) With your left index or middle finger at the back of the articular pillar of her C4, lift her head with both your hands until you feel the tension just reach C4. The finger for this purpose is on the articular pillar of the upper vertebra in order to encourage flexion.

(d) With your right hand on the right side of her head, introduce sidebending and rotation to the left until you feel the tension reach the C4 level.

(e) Ask the patient to make a gentle effort to sidebend to the right *or* to attempt to extend her head gently. If extension is to be the effort, the fingers of your right hand should curl over the front of her chin so that you can resist the effort. Rotation could be used but is more difficult for the operator to control.

(f) After 4 or 5 seconds both relax, but do not lose the position.

(g) When she has relaxed fully (and not before), take up the slack by extension and sidebending to the new barrier.

(h) Repeat steps (e), (f) and (g) three or four times.

(i) Retest.

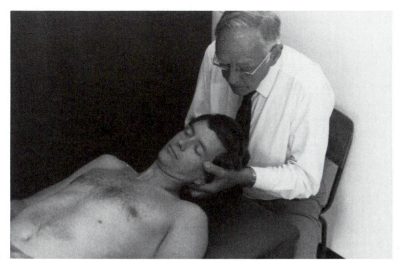

a

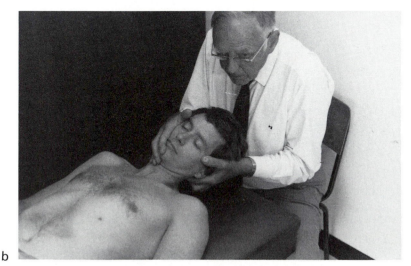

b

Fig. 10.5 Treatment of typical cervical joints (C2–7) for ERS$_R$: **(a)** using sidebend effort, **(b)** using extension effort.

Sitting treatment

These techniques are useful for the lowest cervical joints where the supine techniques are often difficult. They are also good for the T1–2 and T2–3 levels, which may not be easy with the techniques described in Chapter 8.

Technique 6

For restriction of extension. Described for restriction of sidebending and rotation to the left of C7 on T1 (FRS$_R$) (Fig. 10.6).

 1. Diagnostic points.
 (a) In neutral there is some prominence of the right transverse process of C7.
 (b) In extension the relative prominence of C7 on the right is increased.
 (c) In flexion the transverse processes of C7 become even.
 2. Treatment.
 (a) The patient sits with her legs over the side of the table. See that she sits up tall.
 (b) You stand behind her.
 (c) Monitor with your right thumb in contact with the back of the right transverse process of T1 or over the back of the facet joint at C7–T1. It is also possible to use your hands the other way round but the rise in tension of the muscles at your thumb will occur if it is on the side that is made to contract.
 (d) Place your left hand on her head and rotate it to the left up to the barrier.
 (e) Using your right thumb to translate T1 forward to the barrier (as

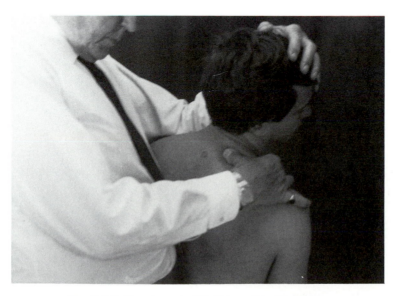

Fig. 10.6 Treatment of C–T junction for FRS$_R$.

well as to monitor) and your left hand to control the head, introduce extension and left sidebending until the tension is felt just to reach the C7 level. The more rotation you have, the less sidebending and/or extension you will need.

(f) Ask her to attempt to move her head into flexion or into right sidebending, or a resultant of the two, while you prevent movement. Rotation can be used but is more difficult to resist. If localisation is correct, you will feel the muscles contract at the right side of the C7–T1 joint.

(g) After 4 or 5 seconds both relax, but do not lose the position.

(h) When she has relaxed fully (and not before), take up the slack in all three directions to the new barrier.

(i) Repeat steps (f), (g) and (h) three or four times.

(j) Retest.

Technique 7

For restriction of flexion. Described for restriction of sidebending and rotation to the left of C7 on T1 (ERS$_R$) (Fig. 10.7).

1. Diagnostic points.

(a) In neutral there is some prominence of the right transverse process of C7.

(b) In flexion the relative prominence of C7 on the right is increased.

(c) In extension the transverse processes of C7 become even.

2. Treatment.

(a) The patient sits with her legs over the side of the table. See that she sits up tall.

(b) You stand behind her.

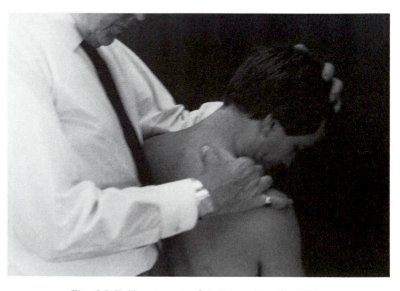

Fig. 10.7 Treatment of C–T junction for ERS$_R$.

(c) Monitor with your right thumb in contact with the back of the right lateral mass of C7. It is also possible to use your hands the other way round but the rise in tension of the muscles at your thumb will occur if it is on the side that is made to contract.

(d) Place your left hand on her head and rotate it to the left up to the barrier.

(e) Using your right thumb to monitor and your left hand to control the head, ask her to slump slightly to allow flexion both below and above C7–T1.

(f) Introduce left rotation and left sidebending until the tension is felt just to reach the C7 level. The more flexion you have, the less sidebending and/or rotation you will need.

(g) Ask her to attempt to move her head into extension or into right sidebending, or a resultant of the two while you prevent movement. Rotation can be used but is more difficult to resist.

(h) After 4 or 5 seconds both relax, but do not lose the position.

(i) When she has relaxed fully (and not before), take up the slack in all three directions to the new barrier.

(j) Repeat steps (g), (h) and (i) three or four times.

(k) Retest.

Semispecific treatment

Like the other semispecific treatments described, these are high velocity thrusting procedures. Perhaps even more than in other regions, it is important to emphasise the *low amplitude* part of the description. One of the authors (JFB) used to use this technique regularly, even at the C1–2 joint, but he now very rarely uses it above about the C4 level (see the warning at the head of this chapter). There are many other thrusting techniques for the cervical region but this author's experience suggests that this is one of the least uncomfortable for the patient.

Technique 8

It will be described for restriction of motion at C5–6, with maximum tissue tension on the left side (Fig. 10.8).

1. The patient sits on the table with her legs over the side. For a short operator with a tall patient it may be easier if she sits on a stool. See that she sits up tall.

2. You stand in front of her.

3. Put your right middle (or index) finger around the left side of her neck so that the terminal phalanx hooks over the spinous process of C5 and the proximal interphalangeal joint comes over the lateral mass of the same vertebra. (See note below.)

4. With your left hand, hold the right side of her head.

5. Monitor with your right finger while you adjust the position of her head to bring the tension to that finger. This will require sidebending to the left (your right) and either flexion or extension. It is usual to find

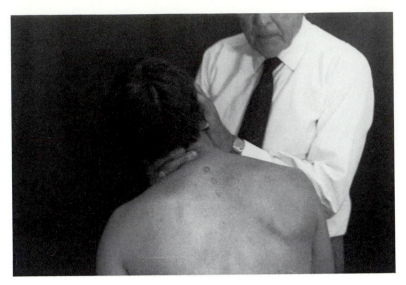

Fig. 10.8 Semispecific high velocity treatment for
C3 to T1, shown for hypertonus on the left at C5–6.

that either flexion or extension will bring the tissue tension to a point
where you meet a barrier, while in the other direction there is no such
feeling.

6. Add rotation as the final movement, using your right finger to pull
on C5 and your left hand to turn her head in the same direction (to
the right). Like the previous movement, this must not be carried to the
point where the joint is 'locked'.

7. The thrust is given by a short sharp increase in the rotatory pressure
simultaneously with both hands.

8. Retest.

Note. For C7 and T1 and, in some patients, for C6, one's middle finger
is not long enough to reach to the other side of the spinous process.
For these levels you should contact the back of the lateral mass of C6
or 7 or the transverse process of T1 with the terminal phalanx of the
finger. The support of the index finger applied to the nail of the middle
finger then helps.

Chapter 11

The Thoracic Cage

The proper functioning of both the respiratory and circulatory systems depends on the integrity and mobility of the chest. The ribs and inter-costal muscles are the structures that preserve the integrity of the chest and their primary function is to allow the creation of a negative pressure inside the chest, which is necessary for inhalation and for both venous and lymphatic return. In addition, the lower ribs are points of origin for the diaphragm and its action can be adversely affected by rib dysfunction.

The thoracic inlet is known to be important because in some circum-stances the thin walled structures which pass through it can be partially obstructed. Dysfunction in this area can be of great significance. The thoracic inlet is bounded by the manubrium sterni in front, the first rib on either side and the body of the first thoracic vertebra behind. The second ribs are also important because of the effect they can have on the mechanics of the sternum.

To the DO the concept that dysfunction of structures in this area could produce enough disturbance in the vessels to be a cause of symptoms is nothing new. To the MD the idea is likely to seem strange, but there is no doubt that the results of accepting the concept and treating accord-ingly are real and helpful.

The location of the sympathetic chain ganglia lying, as they do, just anterior to the costovertebral joints offers a possible explanation for the known sympathetic disturbances that can be associated with dysfunction of the joints of the thoracic cage. This applies with particular force to the stellate ganglion because of the frequency of dysfunction of the first rib and the C7–T1–T2 segments.

RESPIRATORY RIB DYSFUNCTIONS

In certain circumstances rib motion can be restricted so that the excur-sion on inhalation or that on exhalation is limited. This is often associ-ated with thoracic joint dysfunction at the same level but will not necessarily be corrected when the thoracic joint is treated. These restric-tions are known as respiratory rib dysfunctions. The restriction is most easily seen by observing which side stops moving first when the patient takes a full inhalation (or exhalation). Assessment of the difference in the range of movement on the two sides is more difficult.

The ribs move in inhalation so that both the anteroposterior and the lateral diameters of the chest are enlarged. Based on the analogy of the old long handled kitchen pump, the former movement is known as pump-handle, the latter as bucket-handle motion. All ribs have some element of both pump- and bucket-handle motion. The amount of each depends on the obliquity of the line between the costovertebral and costotransverse joints. The higher ribs have more pump-handle and the lower ones, down to 10, have more bucket-handle motion. The 11th and 12th ribs, which have neither costal cartilage nor costotransverse joint, behave more simply. Their movement is described as being like that of calipers.

If on examining the chest for movement one finds more restriction in the bucket-handle mode, the correction should be designed to treat this in preference. Similarly, if the major restriction is of pump-handle movement, the treatment ought primarily to address that mode. It is of greater importance to treat the correct phase of respiration.

When there is restriction of inhalation, the most important, or 'key', rib is the uppermost restricted one. The next lower ribs are prevented from moving normally by the obstruction caused by the upper one. If the uppermost restricted rib is treated, the lower ones will usually be found to move freely again. Occasionally there is a second rib that needs treatment. In restriction of exhalation it is the lowest restricted rib that is the key and it should always be treated first.

STRUCTURAL RIB DYSFUNCTIONS

When the thoracic joints are dysfunctional there can be a disturbance in the shape of the costovertebral joints. This can make the rib either subluxate or twist. The subluxation is a small movement, the joint is not disrupted. The rib head can move either forward (and medially) or backward and laterally. Torsion can also occur and is most common with thoracic joint dysfunction in which there is type II restriction of flexion with loss of sidebending and rotation to the same side. The side to which the joint is sidebent is the one usually affected.

Subluxation of the costovertebral joint of the first rib can also occur. It is often the result of scalene muscle overaction secondary to trouble in the intervertebral joints in the immediate area.

Rib torsion is always associated with type II dysfunction of the corresponding spinal joint. If there is an ERS lesion, the rib torsion on that side will be external; with an FRS lesion the torsion would be internal.

The rib subluxations and torsions are usually known as **structural** rib dysfunctions. They are always associated with thoracic joint problems and will often be corrected when the thoracic joint is successfully treated. They are almost always accompanied by more or less severe pain. There will also be restriction of respiratory movement.

Rib subluxations are relatively common in road accidents. They occur most frequently at the T4 to T7 levels.

It is important to treat any structural rib dysfunctions before the respiratory restrictions are dealt with. Therefore the order of treatment in this region should be the intervertebral joints first, because many structural rib problems will thereby be corrected, any remaining structural rib problems second and, finally, the respiratory restrictions.

Diagnosis

1. To find restriction of rib motion.

(a) The patient lies supine.

(b) You stand to the side which most easily puts your master eye over the midline of her body.

(c) With your hands roughly parallel, place the tips of your index fingers on the anterior ends of her first ribs immediately distal to the inner end of the clavicle (Fig. 11.1). It is possible to put the tips of your middle fingers on the second rib on either side and the ring finger on the third.

(d) Some examiners prefer to place the palm of the hand over the anterior ends of the upper ribs and to feel with the whole hand. If the whole hand is used, it is important that the pressure exerted should be uniform over the area. Pressure, in any case, must be very light or it may interfere with the movement.

(e) Ask her to inhale deeply while you watch to see which side stops moving first. Observe whether the restriction is at the first rib or only lower.

(f) Then ask her to exhale fully and again observe which side stops moving first. If you wish to repeat the tests more than once, it is kind to avoid making the patient breathe deeply, both in and out, too many times because of the discomfort of acapnia. This can be avoided if you observe in the first two breaths which is the restricted phase. If inhalation is restricted, she should breathe out only part way and then take a deep

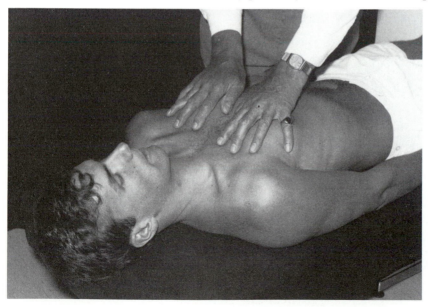

Fig. 11.1 Examination for respiratory restriction in upper three ribs.

breath in. Similarly for exhalation. In exhalation, the key rib is the lowest one showing restriction of movement.

(g) Having tested the upper three ribs, move your fingers down to the next four (using the fifth finger as well) and repeat the examination in both inhalation and exhalation. To assess pump-handle motion, the fingers need to be near the anterior ends of the ribs, for bucket-handle motion they should be more lateral (Fig. 11.2).

(h) Once again, move down to assess the 8th, 9th and 10th ribs by the same method. For the lower ribs the fingers should be in the axilla in order to pick up the main movement, which is of the bucket-handle type.

(i) For the lowest two ribs the patient should be prone (Fig. 11.3). Find the ribs near their inner ends, then move your fingers along the ribs to the anterior end and assess the movement on respiration in the same way. Subluxations do not occur in the lowest two ribs.

2. To find subluxations and torsions of ribs.

(a) The presence in the thoracic spine between T4 and T8 of a joint with restriction of flexion and of sidebending to the same side as rotation should alert the examiner to the possible existence of a structural rib lesion, the more so if there is chest wall pain.

(b) The most important landmark is the rib angle. The line of the rib angles from above down forms a smooth curve, diverging from the midline as the rib number increases. The angle is the site of attachment of the iliocostalis muscle. In most people it can be felt without difficulty. The inner end of the posterior rib shaft is directed posterolaterally from the costovertebral joint to the costotransverse joint. The axis of movement of the rib passes in front of the angle and it is important to remem-

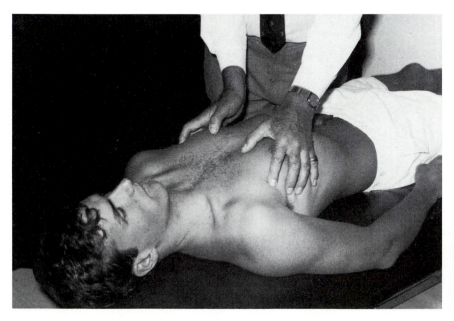

Fig. 11.2 Examination for respiratory restriction in lower ribs.

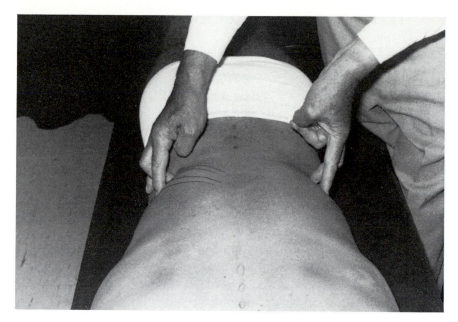

Fig. 11.3 Examination for respiratory restriction in ribs 11 and 12.

ber that when the anterior end of the rib goes up in inhalation, the angle goes down.

(c) If the patient is sitting, she must 'sit up tall' and bring her shoulders forwards. If prone, she should have her head central (not turned to one side) and her arms should drop over the sides of the table. If the table is wide, it may not be possible to get the scapulae out of the way, and the sitting position must then be used. The scapula covers several rib angles when in the adducted position.

(d) In a rib subluxation, the rib angle will be found out of the smooth curve. In a posterior subluxation the obliquity of the line of movement brings the rib angle laterally. In an anterior subluxation it moves medially. In an anterior subluxation the angle will be depressed and the costochondral junction will be prominent. In a posterior subluxation the reverse is true, the angle is prominent and the costochondral junction depressed. There will be tenderness at the angle in any subluxation and often in the intercostal muscles as well.

(e) In a torsion there will also be tenderness at the angle but the curve will not usually be distorted. The diagnosis is made by finding that the rib shaft is twisted. The intercostal space above is not the same width as that below, and one margin of the rib is sharper than the other. If the rib is twisted out (external torsion), the upper margin will be sharp and the lower rounded and the space above will be wider than the space below. In internal torsion the lower space will be the wider and the lower margin the sharp one.

TREATMENT OF THORACIC CAGE DYSFUNCTION

As outlined above, the normal order in which the structures of the thoracic cage should be treated is:

1. thoracic intervertebral joints, including, if indicated, the C7–T1 level (described in Chapters 8, 9 and 10);
2. structural rib dysfunctions;
3. respiratory rib dysfunctions.

Structural rib dysfunctions

Subluxation of the first rib

This is different from ribs 2 to 10 in many respects. For the present purpose, the differences that are important are that there is only a single facet on the rib head for articulation with T1 and that the powerful scalene muscles can pull the rib up into superior subluxation. There can also be an element of either anterior or posterior subluxation.

Much of the rib is covered by the clavicle and crossed by nerves of the brachial plexus and by vessels on their way to the axilla. Because of the sensitivity of these structures, it is important to handle the rib gently and, as far as possible, out of the way of the nerve trunks.

In spite of the fact that intervertebral dysfunction cannot affect the shape of the vertebral component of the costovertebral joint, it is found that it is most important to correct intervertebral joint dysfunction at this level before treating the rib joints.

1. Diagnosis.
(a) Pain locally and referred to arm, neck or head.
(b) Restricted motion of the rib in inhalation, exhalation or both.
(c) Palpable displacement of the inner part of the rib at the back. In superior subluxation the head of the rib will be found to be as much as 4–6 mm (0.16–0.25 inch) higher than on the normal side.
(d) The presence of a dysfunction of the C7–T1 or T1–2 joints, which must be treated first.
2. Treatment (described for the right side) (Fig. 11.4).
(a) The patient sits on a table or stool.
(b) You stand behind her and put your left foot on the seat beside her in order to support her under her left axilla. In this position, sideways movement of your left knee can be used to control her trunk position.
(c) Use your left hand on her head to sidebend her neck to the right without any rotation.
(d) With the fingers of your right hand, lightly palpate the rib in front of the trapezius. With your right thumb, find the posterior aspect of the rib through the trapezius.
(e) Adjust the position of the head and neck to give maximum relaxation and, with your left leg, adjust the trunk position to keep her in balance in the new position.

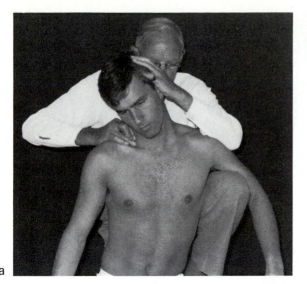
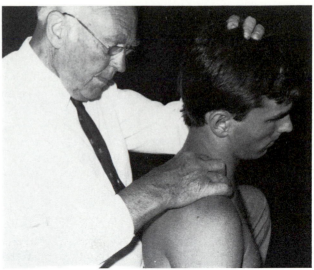

a
b

Fig. 11.4 (a) and **(b)** Treatment of superior subluxation of right 1st rib.

(f) Ask her to push her head to the left with not more than moderate force while you resist. You should not allow movement to occur. This is done in order to secure as much relaxation of muscle on the right side as possible by reciprocal inhibition. If the patient pushes too hard, the muscles on the right side will tighten again and make correction almost impossible.

(g) When the muscles are relaxed, you gently guide the rib head back into position. To bring the rib posteriorly, the shaft should be brought laterally in relation to the transverse process of T1. To correct a posterior subluxation, the rib must be moved medially. If it is superior, it may need to be moved anterolaterally before it will move down; it can 'hitch' on the top of the transverse process.

(h) As is true of all rib subluxations, reduction may require more than one attempt.

Posterior subluxation of ribs 2 to 10

1. Diagnosis.
(a) The level is probably between T4 and T10 and, until it was treated, there was probably a type II restriction at the intervertebral joint with loss of flexion.
(b) The rib angle is lateral to the line of the other angles.
(c) The insertion of iliocostalis at the angle is tender.
(d) The rib angle is posterior, as is the costochondral junction.
(e) Posterior subluxation can only occur if the rib also moves laterally.
2. Treatment (described for the right side) (Fig. 11.5).
(a) The patient sits on a stool or with her legs over the side of the table.

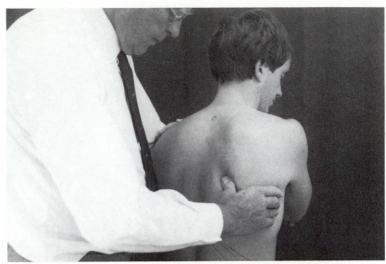

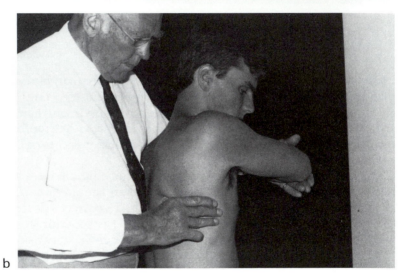

Fig. 11.5 (a) and **(b)** Treatment of posterior subluxation of a right rib.

(b) You stand behind her.

(c) Place your right thumb on the shaft of the rib lateral to the angle.

(d) Ask her to put her right hand on her left shoulder.

(e) Reach round her with your left hand and grip her right elbow
so that you can resist her movement.

(f) While you push medially and forwards with your thumb on her
rib, she should attempt to push her elbow to the left side or to raise
it forwards against your resistance.

Anterior subluxation of ribs 2 to 10

1. Diagnosis.

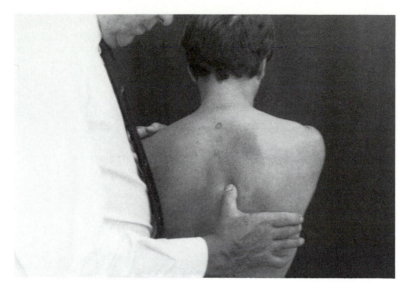

Fig. 11.6 Treatment of anterior subluxation of a right rib.

(a) The level is probably between T4 and T10 and, until it was treated, there was probably a type II restriction at the intervertebral joint with loss of flexion.

(b) The rib angle is medial to the line of the other angles.

(c) The insertion of iliocostalis at the angle is tender.

(d) The rib angle is anterior, as is the costochondral junction.

(e) Anterior subluxation can only occur if the rib also moves medially.

2. Treatment (described for the right side) (Fig. 11.6).

(a) The patient sits on a stool or with her legs over the side of the table.

(b) You stand behind her.

(c) Place your right thumb on the shaft of the rib medial to the angle.

(d) Ask her to put her right hand on her left shoulder.

(e) Reach round her with your left hand and grip her right elbow so that you can resist her movement.

(f) While you pull laterally with your thumb on her rib, she should attempt to pull her elbow to the right side or downwards, or you put your left fist in front of the rib so that when she tries to pull her forearm down towards her she will push your fist and the rib backwards.

Rib torsions

1. Diagnosis.

(a) The level is usually between T4 and T10 and, until it was treated, there was probably a type II dysfunction at the intervertebral joint with restriction of flexion if there is external torsion and restriction of extension if the torsion is internal.

(b) The insertion of iliocostalis at the angle is tender.

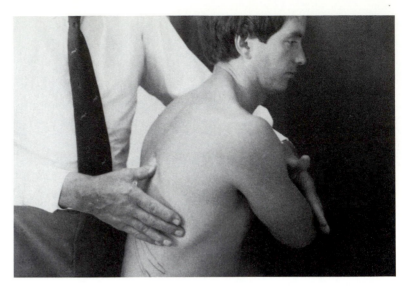

Fig. 11.7 Treatment of external torsion of a right rib.

(c) In external torsion, the intercostal space above is wide and that below is narrow. In internal torsion, the reverse is true.

(d) In external torsion, the upper margin of the rib is sharp and the lower margin rounded. In internal torsion, the lower margin is sharp and the upper rounded.

2. Treatment of external torsion, muscle energy technique (described for the right side) (Fig. 11.7).

(a) The patient sits on a stool or with her legs over the side of the table.

(b) You stand behind her.

(c) Place your right thumb on the under part of the angle of the rib so that pressure upwards will tend to roll the rib into internal rotation.

(d) Ask her to put her right hand on her left shoulder.

(e) Reach round her with your left hand and grip her right elbow so that you can resist her movement. Bring her elbow so that it is almost directly in front of the rib angle, until you feel the beginning of movement of the rib.

(f) Ask her to attempt to raise her right elbow against your resistance while you roll the rib angle up and forwards.

3. Treatment of external torsion and of the spinal joint dysfunction by a combined high velocity technique. Described for restriction of flexion and of left rotation and sidebending (ERS$_R$ at T8–9 with external torsion of the right 8th rib (Fig. 11.8)).

(a) The patient lies on her back.

(b) You stand on her left (contrast Chapter 8, technique 10a).

(c) Ask her to cross her arms over her chest with the right elbow anterior and her hands in her axillae.

(d) Lift her right shoulder with your right hand so that you can insert your left hand under her at the T9 level.

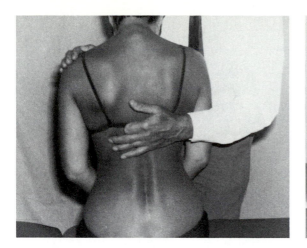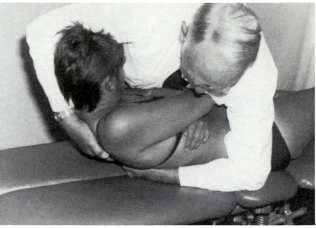

Fig. 11.8 Combined high velocity treatment of ERS$_R$ at T8–9 with external torsion of the right 8th rib.

(e) Your left index finger should be fully flexed at the interphalangeal joints and is used to contact the left transverse process of her T9 (the more posterior at that level).

(f) Bring your left thenar eminence into contact with the inferior edge of the shaft of her right 8th rib medial to the angle.

(g) Allow her trunk to return to the table with your hand underneath.

(h) Slide your right hand down under her head and neck to reach the upper thorax and use it to introduce flexion, left rotation and left sidebending down to T8 while you monitor with your left hand.

(i) The correction is made by a midline downward thrust on her elbows, given with your chest. At the same time you supinate your left hand so that the angle of the rib is lifted craniad to correct the torsion.

(j) Retest.

4. Treatment of internal torsion (described for the right side) (Fig. 11.9).

(a) The patient sits on a stool or with her legs over the side of the table.

(b) You stand behind her.

(c) Place your right thumb on the upper part of the angle of the rib so that pressure downwards will tend to roll the rib into external rotation.

(d) Ask her to put her right hand on her left shoulder.

(e) Reach round her with your left hand and grip her right elbow so that you can resist her movement. Bring her elbow so that it is almost directly in front of the rib angle, until you feel the beginning of movement of the rib.

(f) Ask her to attempt to pull her right elbow down against your resistance while you roll the rib angle downwards and forwards.

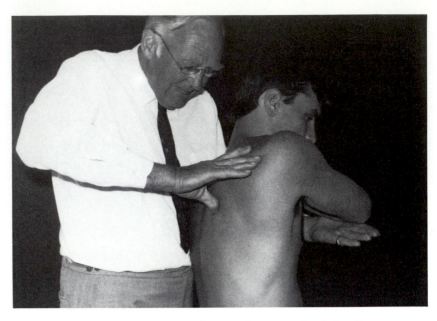

Fig. 11.9 Treatment of internal torsion of a right rib.

Respiratory rib dysfunctions

Inhalation restrictions

1. Diagnosis.
(a) On inhalation, the ribs stop moving earlier on one side than on the other.
(b) Find the uppermost (key) restricted rib.

Technique 1

Muscle energy treatment of inhalation restriction of ribs 1 and 2 (described for the right side). Isotonic contraction of the scalenes is used to raise the front of the ribs at the end of inhalation while you assist with downward pressure on the rib angles to elevate the front (Fig. 11.10).

1. The patient lies on her back.
2. You stand on her left. Lift her right shoulder with your right hand and insert your left hand under her upper back so that you can hook the tips of your index and middle fingers over the inner shafts of her first and second ribs.
3. Allow her right shoulder to return to the table.
4. Turn her head to the left and place her right forearm over her forehead with her elbow at a right angle. (If she has a stiff right shoulder, the forearm placement can be omitted.)
5. Place your right hand on her left forearm (or forehead).

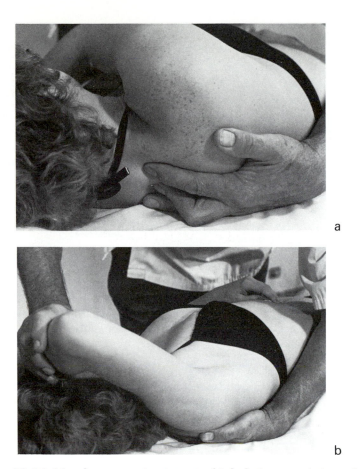

Fig. 11.10 Muscle energy treatment of inhalation restriction of right 1st and 2nd ribs: **(a)** position of fingers, **(b)** position for effort.

6. Ask her to inhale deeply and then lift her head, and forearm, against the resistance of your right hand while, with your left two fingers, you pull laterally and caudad on the back of her first two ribs.

7. Relax, take up the slack by pulling with your left fingers and repeat two or three times and then retest.

Technique 2

Muscle energy treatment of inhalation restriction of ribs 3, 4 and 5 (described for the right side). Isotonic contraction of the pectoralis minor at the end of inhalation is used to raise the front of the ribs while you use downward pressure on the rib angles to assist (Fig. 11.11).

1. The patient lies on her back.

2. You stand on her left. Lift her right shoulder with your right hand and insert your left hand under her upper back so that you can hook the tips of your index, middle and ring fingers over the inner shafts of her 3rd, 4th and 5th ribs.

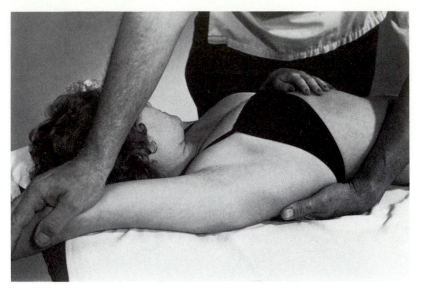

Fig. 11.11 Muscle energy treatment of inhalation restriction of right ribs 3, 4 and 5, for pump-handle dysfunction.

3. Allow her right shoulder to return to the table.

4. For a pump-handle restriction, raise her right arm so that it lies on the table beside her head.

5. If the restriction is more of the bucket-handle type, the starting position of her right arm should be changed. The muscle pull is more effective if her arm points upwards and away from her trunk at about 30°.

6. With your right hand on her right arm just above the elbow, resist her effort while she tries to bring the arm forward (raise it towards the ceiling). This is done when she has taken a deep breath in and, at the same time, you pull caudad and laterally with your left fingers on the back of her ribs.

7. If she has a stiff right shoulder, use your right thumb to contact the coronoid process of her right scapula; take up the slack by upward pressure on the coronoid and her effort should then be to pull the coronoid downward and medially.

8. Relax, take up the slack by pulling with your left fingers and repeat two or three times and then retest.

Technique 3

Muscle energy treatment of inhalation restriction of ribs 6 to 10 (described for the right side). Isotonic contraction of the serratus anterior and pectoralis major is used to raise the front of the ribs while you use respiration and downward pressure on the rib angles to assist (Fig. 11.12).

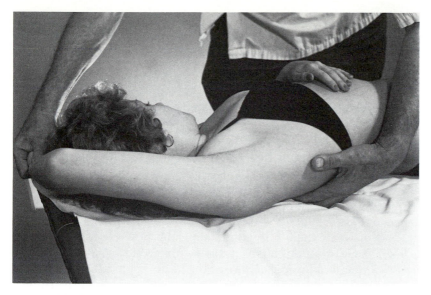

Fig. 11.12 Muscle energy treatment of inhalation restriction of right ribs 6 to 10.

1. The patient lies on her back.
2. You stand on her left. Lift her right shoulder with your right hand and insert your left hand under her back so that you can hook the tips of your four fingers over the inner shafts of her lower ribs. Four ribs can be treated at once, remembering that in restriction of inhalation, the uppermost restricted rib is the key.
3. Allow her right shoulder to return to the table.
4. Raise her right arm so that it lies on the table beside her head. This time she should bend her right elbow so that her forearm lies above her head. Hold her right wrist with your right hand so that you will be able to resist her effort.
5. Ask her to inhale deeply and then attempt to pull her right arm to the right while you resist, and also pull caudad and laterally on the angles of her ribs with your left fingers.
6. If her right shoulder is stiff, you can reach round her with your right hand and press against the lateral border of her right scapula. Her effort then should be to pull her shoulder forwards.
7. Relax, take up the slack by pulling with your left fingers and repeat two or three times and then retest.

Exhalation restrictions

1. Diagnosis.
(a) On exhalation, the ribs stop moving earlier on one side than on the other.
(b) Find the lowest (key) restricted rib.

Technique 4

Muscle energy treatment of exhalation restriction of the first rib. Described for the right side (Fig. 11.13): 'the disappearing thumb trick'.

1. The patient lies on her back.
2. You stand at her head and lift it with your left hand.
3. For the more common pump-handle restriction, you position her head by flexion and right sidebending of her neck. This will relax her muscles and allow you to slide your right thumb *gently* down onto the anterior end of her right first rib. This you will find just behind and below the medial end of her right clavicle.
4. For the bucket-handle restriction, the position requires more sidebending and the thumb makes contact with the shaft of the rib *behind the neurovascular bundle*.
5. Ask her to exhale fully and follow the downward movement of the first rib with your thumb. At the same time you can help by increasing the forward and right sidebending of the neck.
6. Ask her to relax and inhale partially while you hold the rib down to the point it had reached.
7. Repeat the exhalation procedure and subsequent relaxation two or three times.
8. Finally, ask her to attempt to force her head back to the table top against your yielding resistance while you hold the rib down. *This is a painful procedure, particularly this last step.*
9. Retest.

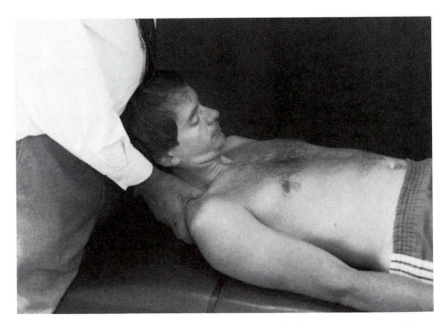

Fig. 11.13 Muscle energy treatment for exhalation restriction of right 1st rib.

Technique 5

Muscle energy treatment of exhalation restriction of ribs 2 to 10. Described for the right side (Fig. 11.14).

1. The patient lies on her back.

2. You stand at her head and, with your left hand, lift her head, neck and the uppermost part of her trunk.

3. While you relax the muscles on the right by flexion and right sidebending of her neck and upper trunk, you place your right thumb and thenar eminence across the costochondral junction of the key rib. It is important to span the costochondral junction as it may otherwise be strained.

4. Ask her to exhale fully and reach down gently with her right hand towards her right knee. At the same time you follow the rib down with your right thumb and increase the movement of her head, neck and upper trunk.

5. For restrictions that are primarily pump-handle in type, you should flex the neck and trunk more than sidebend them. For those that are primarily bucket-handle in type, more sidebending is helpful.

6. Relax, allow her to inhale partially and then repeat the movement two or three times.

7. Finally, ask her to straighten her neck and trunk against your yielding resistance while you hold the rib down in the position that has been achieved.

8. Retest.

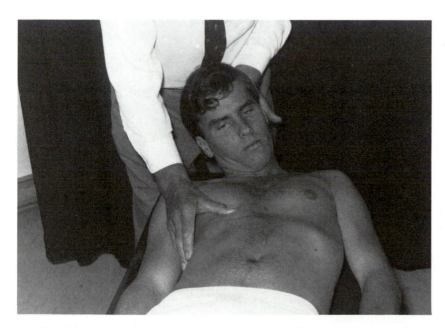

Fig. 11.14 Muscle energy treatment for exhalation restriction of right ribs 2 to 10.

Technique 6

High velocity treatment for respiratory rib dysfunctions. This technique is similar to the supine thoracic techniques described in Chapter 8 as technique 10. The difference is in the placement of the fulcrum and the direction of the thrust.

1. The patient lies on her back.
2. You stand on the side opposite to that to be treated.
3. Ask her to cross her arms over her chest with the arm on the side to be treated in front of the other.
4. With your craniad hand, lift her shoulder on the affected side.
5. Insert your other hand under her in such a way that the spinous processes lie in the hollow of your hand, your fingers supporting the normal side and your thenar eminence in contact with the affected rib close to the angle. For an exhalation restriction, the thenar eminence should be coming up from below the rib; for an inhalation restriction, it should come down from above to contact the upper edge.
6. Allow her trunk to return to the table but use your craniad hand to pull forwards and downwards on her shoulder on the affected side to bring the tissue tension down to the level of the dysfunction.
7. The thrust is given by a sharp increase in downward pressure with your chest over her elbows, directed towards your thenar eminence.
8. Retest.

Respiratory restrictions of the 11th and 12th ribs

The principles are first to disengage the head of the rib and then to use the abdominal muscles as an activating force to move the rib in the only direction available.

Diagnose by finding a restriction of movement on one side on inhalation or exhalation.

Technique 7

Treatment of inhalation restriction (described for the right side) (Fig. 11.15).

1. The patient lies prone.
2. You stand to her left side.
3. Ask her to raise her right arm above her head.
4. With the heel of your left hand, press laterally and slightly craniad on the medial part of the rib.
5. With your right hand, lift her right anterior superior iliac spine off the table.
6. Ask her to make a full inhalation effort and at the same time pull her right hip towards the table against your resistance.
7. Relax, take up the slack with your right hand and then repeat two or three times before retesting.

Technique 8

Treatment of exhalation restriction (described for the right side) (Fig. 11.16).

1. The patient lies prone.
2. You stand to her left side.
3. Ask her to leave her right arm by her side.
4. With the heel of your left hand, press laterally and slightly caudad on the medial part of the rib.
5. With your right hand, lift her right anterior superior iliac spine off the table.
6. Ask her to make a full exhalation effort and at the same time pull her right hip towards the table against your resistance.
7. Relax, take up the slack with your right hand and then repeat two or three times before retesting.

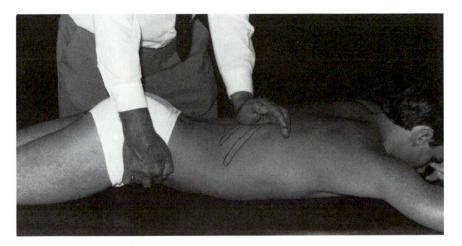

Fig. 11.15 Treatment for inhalation restriction of ribs 11 and 12.

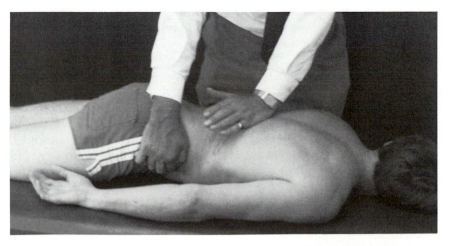

Fig. 11.16 Treatment for exhalation restriction of ribs 11 and 12.

Chapter 12

The Plan of Treatment

THE NATURE OF THE DYSFUNCTION

The findings which are consistently present on examination of those with dysfunction of spinal joints are localised loss of mobility and abnormality of tissue texture. The tissue changes almost always include hypertonus in muscle in the same segment as the loss of mobility. It is worth reiterating that these changes are strictly objective and are therefore of great value in medicolegal cases. It is not possible for someone at will to make a single spinal joint stiff while its neighbours move, and the same is true of the hypertonus and other tissue texture changes.

In the Third Edition of this book, the main emphasis was placed on the hypertonus in muscle as being the chief cause of pain and the reason for the joint stiffness. That concept is useful as a working hypothesis when trying to understand what is happening in the spine, but it is not the whole story. The known effectiveness of muscle energy and, even more so, of indirect techniques lends support to the concept that the soft tissue changes are the most important. On the other hand, there are pointers that this is not the complete answer. At times, during a muscle energy treatment, the joint will suddenly 'let go' with an audible and palpable movement. It is difficult to ascribe the stiffness solely to hypertonus when that happens!

There is a variety of indirect treatments which can be used. Details will not be given in this volume, but to explain the argument the principles of one such treatment will be outlined. The direct action techniques described in these pages all require that the barrier be found and engaged; there are a number of different ways in which the barrier may be overcome.

In the indirect technique sometimes known as **balance and hold**, the dysfunction is approached in a quite different manner. The problem is identified in the usual way but instead of taking the joint up to the barrier, it is taken away. The object of the positioning in this case is to take the joint to the place where the tensions in the tissues around it are balanced in all three planes. The joint is then at the point of maximum ease. This is likely to be near the midpoint of the remaining motion; it will not be in the same place as it would have been if the joint were not restricted. The point of maximum ease must be found accurately by the palpating fingers and, in order to allow this, the patient must be relaxed.

After a short time the point of maximum ease will start to move. The fingers must continue to monitor the tissues all the time and when the beginning of a release is felt, the position should be adjusted so that the joint is moved to its new position of maximum ease. This process is repeated until there is resolution or until no more improvement takes place. The only external force applied is the very gentle movement to adjust the position, and this type of technique can therefore be used in those who are very sick, if for any reason there is an indication to treat their spinal joints.

The mechanism of release is not fully understood but the hypertonus in the muscles can be felt to melt away, and, when it has done so, the pain will be found to have gone or to be much less severe. The fact that this kind of treatment can be effective is a strong argument in favour of the importance of the muscle and other soft tissues as a major part of the cause of the dysfunction.

WHAT IS THE TROUBLE IN THE MUSCLE?

It appears to be an overaction of the gamma motoneuron system which becomes self-perpetuating. When this happens the spindle(s) become shorter and lead to shortening of the whole muscle. If this shortening persists, the muscle cannot relax to its normal resting length.

Such shortening is, of course, physiological. Shortening of the resting length is required prior to certain types of action of muscle, particularly those in which anything near maximum power needs to be exerted through a short range. It is a quite different phenomenon from that of cramp, which appears to be a total contraction of the entire muscle. When the resting length is shortened, the muscle is still able to contract further and then relax back to where it was. It appears that the pain is produced in some way by the muscle's inability to relax to its full resting length.

Even if this is not the whole story, hypertonus of this nature could well be a major part of the cause of the joint stiffness and the associated symptoms. What a pity that the so-called muscle relaxants all seem to be cerebral depressants rather than to have any direct effect on muscle. If some chemical could be found which had a selective effect on the gamma system it might be more helpful, even if it upset the general postural tone of the body.

If one accepts that hypertonus in muscle is a major part of the cause of the dysfunction, why does high velocity manipulation of the joint give relief? It is easier to understand that muscle energy treatment could influence the muscle—isometric exercise has been used for many years to lengthen tight muscle. One of the effects of forced movement of the joint in the right direction is to stretch the muscles by using the bones as levers. This concept could explain the importance of the correct direction for the manipulative movement.

Experience with manipulative treatment shows that it is rarely sufficient to mobilise the affected joint on one occasion only. The muscle appears to behave as if there were a built-in memory in the neuromuscular unit, so that it tends to go back to its contracted state, even when it has been stretched. From the standpoint of neurophysiology, there does not appear to be any reason why the neuromuscular unit should not have a memory of this kind. The number of treatments required varies significantly from patient to patient. The factors which tend to increase the number are the length of time for which the lesion has been present, the violence which produced it, the frequency of similar strains during the course of daily life, and the state of emotional tension of the patient. The last-mentioned will be discussed later.

THE IMPORTANCE OF RE-EXAMINATION

In some patients it is found that the first few manipulations produce a temporary increase in soreness and sometimes also in the total amount of pain. Fortunately, in such cases there is usually some sign of improvement, most commonly an increase in mobility.

A common reason for inadequate improvement following treatment by manipulation is that there has been failure to find the most important joint. Precise diagnosis is not easy. It can become even more difficult if, as a result of overtiredness or for some other reason, the manipulator's sensory perception is not at its best. Errors in precise localisation of the lesion are not uncommon, even among experienced manipulators. Errors can be of two different kinds. In certain circumstances, it is easy to be incorrect in the precise localisation of the signs and to treat the wrong joint. More commonly, the joint which was treated proves to have been of secondary importance only, and the symptoms persist (or even can be aggravated) because the primary joint is still causing trouble. In a patient with pain arising from the low back, there may well be loss of movement and soft tissue changes at the T12–L1 joint, and, indeed, treatment of that joint may be required before the condition is fully resolved. It may be, however, that this same patient has limitation and soft tissue changes in the neighbourhood of the sacroiliac joint. If the sacroiliac joint happens to be the primary cause, treatment at the upper level will at best result in temporary partial improvement. However, treatment of the sacroiliac joint, if it is primary, can even result in resolution of the problem at the upper joint.

The importance of a full structural examination has already been mentioned. These considerations mean that, before each treatment, it is necessary to examine the areas where abnormality has been found. If the condition is unchanged, it suggests that the treatment given was not all that was required. Because of the need to re-examine on each occasion, the authors prefer to do their own treatment rather than delegate it to someone else. In many instances the treatment procedure follows naturally from the examination position and takes very little extra time. If the physician is to delegate treatment, it is essential that the person doing the treatment knows enough to make a confident diagnosis as to the level and direction of the treatment to be given.

TRIGGER POINTS AND AREAS OF
PAINFUL PERIPHERAL MUSCLE

Trigger points

There is one other common cause of persistence of pain in spite of proper manipulative treatment. This is the existence and persistence of secondary areas of painful tight muscle. These used to be known as fibrositis and (even if technically incorrect), when restricted to that meaning, the term was a useful one. These areas are most common in the origin of the two smaller gluteal muscles and in the muscles around the scapula, but they can occur in many other sites. The mechanism of the persistent tightness appears to be a chronic overaction of the gamma system. Travell and others[1-6] have described in beautiful detail a special variety of this more general condition which Travell has called the 'trigger point'.

The true trigger point is specified as predictable in location in any one muscle and as having a predictable pattern of pain reference as well as certain other constant characteristics. The wider areas also tend to cause referred pain, but not necessarily to specific places. Trigger points can occur in any, or almost any, muscle and will often refer pain in other than recognised nerve distributions. The frequent association of both the true trigger point and the wider area of tight muscle with spinal joint dysfunction suggests that the spinal joint dysfunction may be the cause of the peripheral problem. Other possible causes have been suggested by Wyke (see Chapter 13).

Travell lists some of the most common sites for such triggers.

1. Producing pain in the low back:
(a) quadratus lumborum,
(b) longissimus dorsi.
2. Producing pain in the lower limb:
(a) the glutei,
(b) the adductor group.
3. Producing pain in the neck and head:
(a) sternomastoid,
(b) trapezius,
(c) the suboccipital muscles,
(d) the muscles of mastication.
4. Producing pain in the shoulder:
(a) trapezius,
(b) levator scapulae,
(c) the scalenes,
(d) the posterior cervical muscles.
5. Producing pain in the arm:
(a) the spinati,
(b) the scalenes,
(c) deltoid,
(d) subscapularis,
(e) pectoralis major and minor.

The pyriformis should also be mentioned as being important in dysfunction of the pelvic joints. It is also a muscle that is difficult to feel and easy to forget and neglect.

Simons[3] gives an excellent review of the extensive literature on muscle pain syndromes. He credits Reichart as the first, in 1937, to associate explicitly the three classical features:

1. a point of exquisite tenderness within . . .
2. a circumscribed hardening of muscle and
3. pain referred in response to pressure on the tender point.

Travell published her first paper on trigger points in 1942 and has written extensively since then, culminating in the major contribution in collaboration with Simons[6] in 1982, of which the second volume is in preparation. In the meantime Mennell[2,7] has published some of the charts and describes methods of treatment.

Simons[3] points out that the only histological change found (by many investigators) has been mild fibroplasia, and that only in severe long-standing cases. In his conclusion he points out that 'only in the last several decades has the distinction between trigger zones and reference zones been drawn clearly and distinctly'. Reference to the published charts shows that in a few instances the trigger point is actually located inside the reference zone; this, of course, tends to cause confusion. Simons found that 'several lines of evidence have suggested that something interfered with the oxidative metabolism of muscle fibres in the region of a palpable band'.

The precise nature of the changes that cause the thickening and tenderness is still not fully understood but in the minds of many clinicians there is no doubt that such changes exist. Most people who treat musculoskeletal pain will know of patients in whom the treatment of the trigger point resulted in complete relief of the pain. Unfortunately, this is not usually what happens. More commonly, there is temporary relief followed by a return of the pain and, when the pain returns, it will usually be found that the trigger point has once again become active.

It seems that the trigger point in peripheral muscle is itself started by a disturbance of function of its nerve supply. One of the causes of such disturbance of the nerve supply is an interference with normal function in one or more joints in the spine. In those in whom treatment of the trigger point gives lasting relief, it seems reasonable to assume that the original cause is no longer active. In those who get no more than temporary relief from treatment of the trigger point it is likely that there is an active causative lesion elsewhere. Patients coming for treatment of pain should always be checked for the presence of trigger points, but a positive finding does not necessarily complete the diagnosis. It is probably a more common mistake to neglect the trigger points and just treat the spinal joint dysfunction, but it can be equally unsatisfactory to treat the trigger and neglect the spine.

There is an additional reason for finding and treating active trigger points: there appears to be a mechanism whereby an active trigger can, if untreated, result in recurrence of the spinal joint dysfunction which appeared to be its original cause. The mechanism is probably one involving spreading of nerve impulses because the segment has become 'facilitated' by the continuing afferent discharge from the pain-producing lesion. A similar mechanism is likely to be what caused the trigger point in the first place.

Painful areas in peripheral muscle

The painful peripheral muscle areas do not always fit the description of the classical trigger point. For simplicity, these common areas of painful hypertonus will be referred to as 'fibrositis'. They are also associated with referred pain, but of a less predictable pattern. The feeling of these areas on examination is characteristic. Part of the muscle involved feels tight to the fingers and is almost always tender, while the main body of the muscle is soft and relaxed. Maigne has described the feel as being like tight cords when one slides one's finger across the fibres. The impression is of some of the muscle fibres in the area being chronically contracted. That this feeling is not due to fibrosis is shown by the relaxed feel which is apparent immediately after successful treatment.

It is of great importance that one should remember that a referred pain which appears to be exactly the same may on different occasions have different sources. This underlines the importance of a structural examination in every patient to find areas of dysfunction rather than a localised examination of the region from which the symptoms 'ought' to arise. Pain in the lower limb may appear to be exactly the same when it arises from a disturbance of function at L4 and when the cause is a gluteal muscle trigger.

Treatment

Treatment of both the true trigger points and the areas of 'fibrositis' can, of course, be undertaken by a physiotherapist, but fortunately the majority will settle relatively easily, provided that the exciting cause is also treated. The exciting cause is usually a spinal joint dysfunction and it is commonly practicable for the manipulator to treat the peripheral muscle at the same time as he treats the spinal joint. One must not forget, however, that a similar reaction can be produced by other causes of segmental pain, including visceral pathology.

A wide variety of different treatments is available, of which one of the simplest is heat. Heat in any form will do, but dry heat is easier to use than most forms and appears to be as effective. The hot-water bottle and electric hot pad have the advantage that they can be used without the need to undress. The infra-red lamp does not appear to be more efficient and can easily burn the skin if used carelessly, as well as requiring removal of clothing. This treatment can be done by the patient at home. Some favour the use of cold and some patients do say that this form of treatment gives them more relief than does heat. When used as described by Travell and Simons,[6] the cooling is momentary. The cold appears to have the effect of blocking the activity of the gamma motoneurons by the inhibition produced when the alpha fibres are stimulated. When the overactivity of the gamma system is interrupted, it becomes possible to stretch the muscle. Travell strongly advises that the muscle itself should not be chilled as that tends to lead to shivering with further tightening of the muscle fibres.

Massage has been used for the purpose for many years, but in order to be effective it needs to be given deeply. Unfortunately, deep massage over the painful muscle is often acutely painful and it is necessary to start very lightly and gradually increase the depth as the muscle begins to relax. Frictioning with the fingers across the length of the muscle fibres is good if the condition is not too acute. In the most acute, simple pressure followed by gentle rotatory frictioning will sometimes work where anything more energetic would result in generalised spasm. In those in whom even such gentle methods cause too much pain or prove to be ineffective, infiltration of the tender area with 1% local anaesthetic is often very helpful. On no account should the local anaesthetic be mixed with adrenalin because this tends to reproduce the spasm. At one time it was thought that admixture of a steroid was helpful, but this is now considered by many practitioners to be incorrect and the authors no longer use it for this purpose.

Travell has also found that, with the true trigger point, dry needling can result in immediate relaxation and extinguishing of the actual trigger. For this to occur, it is probable that the trigger point must be accurately defined and precisely entered by the point of the needle. It has been claimed that the trigger points are, in fact, acupuncture points but this does not appear to be true of all, although some are very close to classical acupuncture points. The size of the true trigger point is very small, a few millimetres only in the longest diameter.

Travell[5,6] and Mennell[2,7] and their co-workers describe the method of obtaining relaxation of the tight muscle by the use of the vapo-coolant spray. The original method used ethyl chloride, but a mixture of freons has proved to have better characteristics: it is neither inflammable nor explosive, nor is it a general anaesthetic. Almost as important is that the chill produced is less intense. Ethyl chloride chills too much—the object is to stimulate the temperature receptors in the skin, not to chill the muscle. Even when using the freon mixture, care must be taken to see that the deeper tissues are not cooled. The principle is to stretch the muscle during and immediately after the application of the spray and thus to take advantage of the temporary inhibition of the gamma system caused by the activation of the temperature receptors.

Mennell[2,7] gives a series of diagrams covering many of the more common muscles, showing both trigger points and reference zones. Travell and Simons[6] give a comprehensive account of their own and others' work and include detailed instructions as well as diagrams for almost every affected muscle. Other means of applying cold can be used. Dr Audrey Bobb uses ice, but this has the disadvantage that it melts and it is more uncomfortable to use.

If, after treatment, and in particular after injection, a trigger point or an area of painful tight peripheral muscle quickly recurs, it is a sure sign that the causative lesion is still active. In the majority of cases the causative lesion will be a spinal joint that is dysfunctional.

MUSCLE SPASM OVER THE SPINAL JOINT

Treatment is sometimes necessary to the muscles in more immediate relation to the joint at which there is dysfunction. One of the most effective treatments in this situation is massage given transversely, that is, across the muscle fibres which are running up and down the spine. Here again, the massage must be started lightly and slowly. It may be done with the fingertips when it is easier to be on the side being treated. It may also be given with the heel of the hand and in that case it is better to stand on the opposite side and press the muscle mass rhythmically away from the spinous processes. As the tissue relaxes and becomes more mobile the treatment should become deeper. Injections of local anaesthetic may be given into these muscles also and in some instances can be very effective in relieving acute spasm.

EPIDURAL INJECTIONS

An alternative to intramuscular injections of this kind is the caudal epidural route and, when dealing with the low lumbar spine, it is both easy and effective. For this also plain local anaesthetic, used in 0.5% solution, is the agent of choice. When epidural injections are given at the level of the root involved, there is advantage in the use of steroids, but for caudal injections these are not necessary and are better avoided.

The caudal epidural injection is simple and can be done safely in the office. It is most easily given with the patient prone. The sacral hiatus is found and the skin cleansed. The needle should be no longer than 3.8 cm (1.5 inches) so that it is impossible for it to reach the end of the dural sac. There is no need to use a fine needle to anaesthetise the skin, and, after injection of a few drops to lessen the pain, the needle is advanced to the sacral hiatus. The tough fibrous tissue covering the hiatus is recognised and should be penetrated with the needle pointing craniad and forwards at an angle of about 30° to the horizontal. As soon as the needle is through the hiatus, it can be advanced for 13 mm (0.5 inch) or so without difficulty, if correctly placed. The most common mistake is to have the needle pointing too far forwards and to strike the back of the sacral vertebral bodies. After aspirating, to ensure that the needle is not in a vein, the injection can be started. It is uncomfortable in many patients and more so if given fast. If the discomfort becomes severe, it is best to stop for a minute or so until it passes off and then continue. For low lumbar problems, as little as 15 ml will often be enough; if it is necessary to have the effect higher, more will be needed but, in the authors' experience, the very large quantities recommended by Cyriax are not often required.

If the injection is being used to obtain relaxation so that a manipulative procedure can be performed, it is necessary to wait for several minutes to allow diffusion into the nerves to take place. Because of the unlikely possibility that some weakness of the legs might occur during the first 2 hours, it is wise to arrange that the patient has a driver or, alternatively, that she should wait for about 2 hours before driving herself. The patient should also be warned that such weakness, although very unlikely, is a possibility so that she will not be seriously alarmed if it should happen.

The epidural injection of a steroid–local anaesthetic mixture near a nerve root that is inflamed can be very helpful at times, but the authors recommend that this is done in hospital or at a specially equipped clinic. Some workers in this field use 2% saline which, being hypertonic, serves to withdraw fluid from the tissues with which it is in contact. The relief obtained from both steroid and this saline injection does indicate that part of the cause of pain is local inflammation in at least some cases.

MULTIPLICITY OF LEVELS INVOLVED

Experience in a manipulative practice soon shows one that spinal joints which are dysfunctional are rarely single. It would seem 'tidy' to theorise that, when the injury first occurs, only one joint is involved, but there does not appear to be any evidence for that assumption. It is clear that by the time the average patient comes for treatment, a number of joints, and sometimes a large number, are giving trouble. It may be noticed that the authors have accepted in this paragraph that there is an injury to start the problem. This cannot be proved but, if one takes enough trouble with the history, there is nearly always something in the way of an injury, even if it was many years before.

The longer the history since injury, the more likely it is that the dysfunction will be at multiple levels. Often the symptoms appear to arise from one level in particular but, even so, this may not be the most important level. If the level immediately responsible for the symptoms is treated, there is likely to be relief. If, however, this is not the most important joint in the overall picture, the symptoms will soon return, either the same or in a more or less modified form. This is one of the main reasons for performing a thorough structural examination on the first visit and a limited similar examination prior to each treatment.

The human body has a complicated system of positional control so that the head can be held upright and pointing forwards. If there is a mechanical interference with movement at any level, the levels above and below will tend to compensate. If this condition persists, the compensating joint may well become restricted in movement, the more so in the presence of muscle hypertonus. If the first joint is restricted in the right sidebent position, the neighbouring joint will be sidebent left, etc. Some areas of the spine appear to be more liable to develop this secondary stiffness. The regional junctions, where there is a change in mobility and function, are particularly susceptible, as are both ends of the mobile spinal column. Thus one often sees secondary stiffness at the thoracolumbar junction, at the cervicothoracic junction, at the occipitoatlantal joint and in the pelvis. The joint immediately above or below the primary dysfunction may also be affected.

TREATMENT OF A PATIENT WITH A POSSIBLE DISC PROTRUSION

In the absence of signs indicating a space-occupying lesion, it can be very difficult to distinguish, by examination, between a patient with an actual disc protrusion and one with very acute symptoms from a dysfunctional spinal joint without that complication. Experience with manipulative treatment suggests that there is no single clinical sign and no combination of signs that prove diagnostic other than those of a space-occupying lesion. The severity of the pain is no guide, nor is the immobility of the spine, nor the presence of a scoliosis, nor the degree of limitation of straight leg raising, nor the alteration in the straight leg raising test caused by dorsiflexion of the foot. A spinal joint in which disc damage is sufficient for posterior bulging to have started appears not to be made any worse by the type of manipulation described in the earlier chapters. It is often found, however, that the results of manipulation in such cases are less good. The treatment by manipulation can, therefore, be used as a diagnostic test, to be continued only so long as there is continuing improvement.

There is no doubt that the symptoms of some patients with actual disc protrusions do improve with manipulative treatment, although it is usually found that the manipulation is required at some joint other than that at the level of the disc protrusion. In such a case the rate of improvement will often be slower than usual but, as long as improvement is progressive, it is worth continuing unless progress is so slow that it appears that the patient's time is being wasted. If there is doubt as to what is the best approach, it is wise to explain the position in detail to the patient. There are many who will express the wish to avoid surgery if possible and the more so if it is explained that the results of surgery are not always perfect!

It is often forgotten that autopsy examinations sometimes show evidence of old disc protrusions in those for whom no history of back problems can be found. It appears that the softening and subsequent protrusion of disc material is a complication of spinal joint dysfunction but only in some patients does it interfere with recovery enough to justify removal. Chrisman *et al.*[8] report on a series of 38 patients suffering with 'an unequivocal picture of ruptured intervertebral disc unrelieved by conservative care'. Twenty seven of these had positive myelograms. All were submitted to rotatory manipulation under anaesthetic and 20 are reported as having good or excellent results. Ten of those with positive myelograms remained good or excellent 3 years or more after manipulation. The appearance of the myelogram before and after the manipulation, whether positive or negative, was unchanged. They did note, however, that the results were better in the group with negative myelograms.

In the practice of one of the authors (JFB) there was a classical case. A male aged 29, working as a car lease manager, gave a history of intermittent back pain over 2 years which had originally started after a fall. Two months before he was seen he started a fresh attack but this time also had right-sided sciatic pain. He had already spent 3 weeks on traction in hospital with only partial relief and had had a myelogram which showed a filling defect on the right at L5–S1 (Fig. 12.1).

Examination showed marked stiffness of the right sacroiliac joint as well as evidence of dysfunction at other levels, including the lumbosacral joint. As a preliminary, the right sacroiliac joint was treated. There was an almost immediate improvement in the amount of pain and slowly, over about 2 months, the straight leg raising improved also. He received a total of 12 treatments in 2 months but had returned to work after 2 weeks. He came back for two further treatments 3 months later because of a mild recurrence.

The use of epidural steroid injections around a nerve root is established as a valuable adjunct in treatment. It seems that it is particularly indicated in those in whom the pain does not subside in the expected manner when the structural problem has been dealt with. As mentioned earlier, this is better done in a hospital setting by someone familiar with

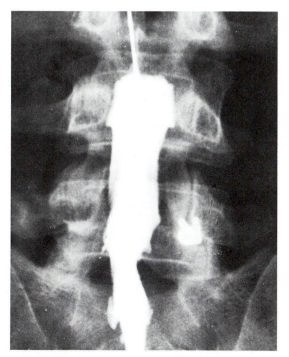

Fig. 12.1 Myelogram showing filling defect on right side at L5–S1.

the technique, and is often performed by those specialising in anaesthesia.

FREQUENCY OF TREATMENT

In any particular patient, the optimum frequency of treatment will depend on a number of factors. If several treatments are given on successive days, there is a danger of a build-up of soreness and it is better to allow a sufficient interval for any reaction to settle. On the other hand, if treatments are spaced too widely, there is a tendency for progress to be too slow. It is wise to try to build on the benefit of one session by treating again before it has vanished. In the experience of one of the authors in a hospital out-patient setting in Britain, it is difficult to arrange for the patients to come back within less than 1 week, but that is much better than waiting 2 weeks unless the majority of the treatment has already been given. Where this is possible, it is better to arrange to see a new patient again after only 1 or 2 days and to continue to treat at less than a week's interval until the condition has begun to show real improvement. It is often a mistake to continue daily treatment for long because of the build-up of soreness.

As soon as real improvement is shown, the frequency of visits is reduced, but it is still important not to make the gap so long that the symptoms have returned in force before another treatment is given. The number of treatments required by patients varies widely. Some, especially those with a fresh injury, may be largely relieved by one treatment. Others may need many. The operator must be guided with respect to the frequency and the number of treatments by his findings on clinical examination. If it is clear that the patient is improving with respect to the extent and intensity of muscle hypertonus and the range of general and specific mobility, then the frequency of treatment can usually be decreased quite rapidly. The large majority of patients will admit to symptomatic improvement corresponding in extent and rate to the observed clinical change. In such patients it is usually safe to allow one's views on frequency and length of treatment to be influenced by their subjective complaints.

The operator is well advised to re-examine carefully any patient in whom improvement is unexpectedly slow. One common cause is that there are one or more other areas of dysfunction which also require treatment. There is also the possibility that there is a visceral condition serving as an irritant to maintain the spinal dysfunction. Mechanical problems in the limbs, especially in the legs, may have a similar effect. The secondary areas of peripheral muscle hypertonus have been discussed above. One other very important cause of slow recovery is discussed in the next section.

THE PROBLEM OF THE NEUROTIC PATIENT

It is well known that back trouble is often found in association with neurosis. In the past this association has proved a particularly tiresome one for the medical practitioner because methods of examining the individual spinal joints have not been taught in the majority of medical schools. Proper assessment of spinal joint problems is very difficult without such examination. Nor is it easy to assess the severity of a neurosis to ascertain if it is bad enough to be the prime cause of the back complaint. There have undoubtedly been many patients whose emotional state has been the basic cause but who have received extensive treatment to their backs because this was the part of which they complained. There are many, however, who show signs of depression or other emotional upset, in whom the back joints are dysfunctional and are the source of their symptoms. The authors have seen and treated successfully many such patients who have often been told by a supposed expert that 'it is all in your head'. It takes a very stable personality not to react emotionally when told that about what appears to be a very genuine physical pain.

This situation is still common because the necessary examination techniques are either not known or not used. It is a very happy moment for patient and physician alike when the clouds lift and a depressed patient becomes normal again, as so often happens in this type of situation when a positive physical diagnosis is made and the patient begins to improve with the treatment.

It would be idle to suggest that the combination does not happen. Indeed it does, and the neurotic with a bad back can be a very difficult and time-consuming problem. If the emotional aspect is largely iatrogenic, from a failure of one or (more commonly) several physicians to find the physical problem, it can be expected to settle as soon as treatment begins to give relief. Unfortunately, there are many patients with genuine somatic dysfunction in spinal joints who also have more or less severe emotional problems, often of a chronic nature.

The patient who presents for examination and in whom there is almost no physical abnormality is relatively easily dealt with. One must, of course, take the trouble to perform a full thorough examination in order to exclude, not only back joint lesions of the type under discussion, but any of the other physical abnormalities that might cause the symptoms. If one has successfully excluded physical causes, the patient should on no account be started on a course of manipulative treatment. Such patients are rare and the following example is a warning to be careful.

A male in his mid-thirties was admitted to an orthopaedic hospital at which, at the time, one of the authors was working. After intensive clinical and x-ray examination he was discharged, labelled as a neurotic, although he was still complaining bitterly of his back. Three months later we heard from a neighbouring hospital that he was dead of leukaemia.

Among those referred for examination because of back complaints the neurotic without back trouble is a comparative rarity. It is much more common to find physical evidence of joint dysfunction, even in those who have an obvious emotional problem. In those in whom the emotional state is a reaction to unrelieved back pain, treatment can proceed as usual, with the expectation of recovery of the emotional problem as the back improves. In others the emotional abnormality can make treatment of the physical problem much more difficult. The effect of emotional tension is well known and many patients already recognise that they are worse when they get worried or angry. Depression has a similar effect, but it is not commonly recognised by the patient. There is evidence[9] that any increase in emotional tension is reflected in the motor activity of the striated muscle throughout the body. It seems reasonable to suggest that, if the tension is increased in a muscle that is already hypertonic, it will increase the tendency of that muscle to cause pain. It also seems that the patient with an emotional upset tends to feel pain more than someone who is relaxed.

In many of these patients, successful treatment of the physical back problem and the elementary psychotherapy which is the stock in trade of any good doctor will help enough and they will get better, even if more slowly than those who are better adjusted. There are some in every practice who are disturbed enough emotionally to make successful treatment almost impossible. It seems that their tensions bring back the physical condition before one has a chance to treat them again. These patients need psychotherapy and it is of great importance that the manipulator should recognise them. If he does not, they will tend to fill his waiting room and bring his practice into disrepute.

DANGERS AND CONTRAINDICATIONS

There is scarcely a treatment in medicine that is without its attendant danger. There is the possibility of doing harm by almost any active treatment, and this is certainly true of manipulation. Fortunately, the danger is small and with care can be avoided. Suitable manipulative procedures are less frequently associated with complications than almost any other treatment. It is of the utmost importance, however, that they should be recognised because, although rare, complications can be serious.

The dangers fall into three groups.

1. Those caused by the manipulation doing damage to a bone weakened by some pathological process, with possible dissemination of that process.

2. Spinal cord or cauda equina pressure caused by a massive disc extrusion.

3. Circulatory disturbance caused by damage to a vessel or by reflex arterial spasm.

Dangers in manipulating a weakened bone

Bone is commonly weakened by one of a few pathological processes. All of these will in time be visible in the x-ray pictures, but patients may well be seen at the stage when the bone is significantly weakened but the x-rays do not yet show any change. This is particularly true of infections and neoplasms. The most common cause of weakening of bone is osteoporosis and this is always detectable in the x-rays.

Clinical judgement is a vital part of the assessment of any candidate for manipulative treatment. The osteoporotic can usually be spotted from across the room if one has a 'high index of suspicion'. No such case should be subjected to high velocity thrusting manipulation without prior radiography. Because the force used in muscle energy treatment is applied by the patient, and for spinal treatment it should always be gentle, this kind of manipulation is considered safe, even in those with moderate loss of bone density.

Many patients with osteoporosis have pain in the back. In some it is the result of vertebral collapse and for them rest for that part of the spine is important. There are many, however, in whom there is no evidence of collapse and the majority of these patients will have the signs of joint dysfunction. Treatment of these joints can be very helpful and need not be withheld because the density of the bones is reduced. Clearly, any high velocity manipulation must be done very gently, but for these patients also muscle energy treatment need not present any hazard.

Tuberculosis is fortunately much less prevalent than formerly. Even so, it remains a danger and one which must not be forgotten because of its comparative rarity. One should be put on one's guard at once because patients with bone or joint infections are ill as well as in pain. The patient with acute back dysfunction is in severe pain but is not 'ill'. A valuable ally is the intensity of the muscle spasm over an infected lesion, quite different from the hypertonus over a dysfunctional joint and much more widespread. Even if an infected bone or joint is mistakenly manipulated, the spasm in the muscles is likely to prevent any damage being done if the force used is no more than that described in the techniques in this volume. This is another good reason for never using a general anaesthetic for this type of treatment. One of the authors had sent to him a man with back pain. He had been treated 21 times in 22 days by a chiropractor whose initial x-rays were reported as normal. There was more spasm than usual and it was on both sides at the same level. Fresh x-rays showed a destructive lesion at L5 which proved to be due to staphylococcal infection. In spite of the number of treatments, there was no clear evidence that the chiropractor had made him any worse; he certainly had not helped!

Simple tumours of sufficient size to weaken the vertebrae are uncommon in the spine.

Primary malignancy is also uncommon, but secondaries are common and may be multiple. A vertebral body may be seriously weakened by a secondary growth before there is any change in the x-ray appearance. Fortunately, the clinical picture will usually point to some major disturbance of the body economy before that stage is reached. If one maintains a high index of suspicion, the clinical picture is likely to alert one to the possibility. This possibility is a good reason for refusing to see a patient unless accompanied by a letter from the family doctor.

Danger of massive disc extrusion

This accident is rare but has occurred often enough to be used as an argument against manipulative treatment.

One author (JFB) has seen two patients to whom it happened—one sat up in bed and coughed, the other bent down to lift a heavy article. Both had recently had treatment by high velocity manipulation with partial relief of symptoms. Both came to surgery and the one for whom the time before surgery was only about 2 hours made a very good recovery. The other did not get to surgery for nearly 24 hours and had residual weakness of his legs.

The only iatrogenic case of which the same author has personal knowledge occurred when the lumbar spine was manipulated under general anaesthetic and the manipulation included flexion. It appears that the type of change in the disc which makes this accident possible is quite uncommon. There must be a separated fragment of sufficient size to cause compression of the cauda equina and, even if not calcified, it must be of firm consistency. As far as the authors are aware, this accident can only happen if there is forced flexion.

If by any chance a massive extrusion does occur with paralysis, exploration and removal of the extruded material are essential and *of extreme urgency*.

Danger of reflex arterial spasm

By far the greatest number of complications of spinal manipulation have arisen following high velocity manipulation of the upper cervical joints. The complication has been virtually confined to the vertebral and basilar arteries and their immediate branches. Those initially drawn to the attention of one of the authors (JFB) were in chiropractors' cases, but in a chapter on *Complications and Contraindications*, Kleynhans[10] gives figures which include 26 cases from chiropractors, 10 from medical manipulators and 14 from Germany where there were a number of physicians using chiropractic-type manipulations. It is interesting that he also lists 8 cases of what he calls 'spontaneous or self-inflicted vertebral artery accidents'. Most of the latter involved sustained extension of the head on the neck with or without rotation of the head.

The anatomy of the vertebral artery is such that in full extension of the head on the neck, if rotation is introduced, the artery is narrowed on the side away from which the face is turned. The narrowing may be enough to cause complete obstruction to the flow of blood. (See Tissington Tatlow and his co-workers,[11,12] who also showed that the application of traction in the cadaver increased the proportion of those with complete obstruction from 4 out of 41 to 17 out of 41.)

Maigne[13] quotes angiographic studies in the living which also sometimes demonstrate complete occlusion. Sheehan *et al.*[14] found that rotation and hyperextension of the neck reproduced the symptoms in those suffering from spondylotic vertebral artery compression, but they thought that the obstruction occurred at the sites of exostoses in the intraforaminal portion of the artery.

It is well known that the vertebral arteries are often asymmetrical in size even when not obstructed in any way. The mechanism of the injury is thought to be a severe reduction in the blood flow on the side with a big artery so that there is insufficient from the narrow vessel on the open side. Transient ischaemia is of little importance and a test has been described to detect those who might be susceptible to this kind of injury. The test involves putting the head in the position which reduces the blood flow unilaterally and watching for nystagmus. *Unfortunately the test itself cannot be regarded as safe. It should **not** be used.* Reference to the mechanisms of injury in the spontaneous group referred to above[10] shows that serious results can follow simple positioning.

The serious results appear all to be due to thrombosis occurring in an artery obstructed mechanically or by spasm. In some series there has been a high percentage of permanent disability or death.

The iatrogenic cases all appear to have occurred during (or immediately after) high velocity manipulation of the occipitoatlantal or atlantoaxial joints. Fortunately, both these joints will almost always respond to muscle energy treatment and this has never been reported as being associated with this complication. The authors no longer feel justified in including descriptions of techniques of high velocity manipulation for these joints, although they are aware that this is still done by many manipulators.

OSTEOARTHRITIS AND SPONDYLOSIS

True osteoarthritis of the apophyseal joints is relatively uncommon and must be distinguished from degenerative disc disease. Osteoarthritis is a disease of diarthrodial joints and the term is incorrect if applied to the spurring and narrowing of disc spaces which is so common and is properly termed degenerative disc disease or spondylosis. The narrowing is the result of the slow absorption of softened disc material and the spurring is probably nature's attempt to limit the abnormal movement which tends to occur when the disc fails to provide its shock-absorbing and fulcrum functions. Both are thought to be late results of injury to spinal joints and are thought not to be visible for about 5 years after the injury which caused the changes. In most cases in the authors' practices, the spurs do *not* indicate the level from which the symptoms arise but only the level of one of the old injuries.

The presence of spurs from spondylosis, even if they are very big ones, is of itself no contraindication to treatment by manipulation, nor do they stop it being effective. The association of severe spondylosis in the neck with a neurological deficit suggesting spinal cord damage is certainly a contraindication to high velocity treatment in that region but judicious use of muscle energy treatment may be helpful.

In the presence of marked spondylotic changes in any region, it is wise to examine carefully the neighbouring regions for unexpected sources of paradoxical referred pain. Patients with pain in the neck and one or both arms will very commonly respond to treatment to the dysfunctional upper thoracic joints even when the cervical joints themselves are stiff and spondylotic.

True osteoarthritis of the facet joints is not necessarily associated with symptoms and, in many patients who show these x-ray changes, symptoms will be found to be arising from other levels. Facet osteoarthritis does not appear to be a contraindication to treatment of dysfunctional joints even by high velocity manipulation.

THE PROBLEM OF THE SHORT LEG

When a patient first presents and is found to have a short leg, it is as well to remember that, unless she has had a recent fracture, the difference has been there all her life and she will be compensated in part at least.

When the right leg is shorter than the left, it is usual to find the left innominate in the posterior position and the right anterior, because that helps to level the sacral base. This, in turn, will cause a rotation of the lower lumbar vertebrae. Either of these asymmetries may become 'fixed' and the cause of symptoms. Observation of leg length disparity is therefore pertinent to one's assessment of the patient.

Many patients with differences of less than 13 mm (0.5 inch) will respond well to treatment of the dysfunctional joints without recourse to heel lifts. In those in whom response is slow or in whom recurrences occur after only a short time, it is often helpful for them to use a raise. If it is decided to use a raise, it is useful to have an accurate measurement of the difference, and methods of doing this are discussed in Chapter 3.

If a raise is prescribed, it is enough for it to be in the heel only, unless the difference is more than 13 mm (0.5 inch). For women's high heels, the heel on the long leg side may be reduced. Movable lifts inside the shoe are not recommended, they move out of position, get lost or get forgotten, and the actual heel should be altered. The amount of the raise should always be a little less than the actual difference in length. It is sometimes recommended to raise the heel in small increments but this is probably an unnecessary complication (and expense!) for the patient.

Lift therapy is discussed in detail by Greenman.[15]

REFERENCES

1. Travell J., Rinzler S. H. (1952). The myofascial genesis of pain. *Postgrad. Med*; 11:425–434.
2. Mennell J. M. (1975). The therapeutic use of cold. *J.A.O.A*; 74:1146–1158.
3. Simons D. G. (1975). Muscle pain syndromes. *Am. J. Phys. Med*; 54:289–311, 55:15–42.
4. Travell J. (1960). Temporomandibular joint dysfunction. *J. Prosthetic Dentistry*; 10:745–763.
5. Travell J. (1952). Ethyl chloride spray for painful muscle spasm. *Arch. Phys. Med*; 33:291–298.

6. Travell J., Simons D. G. (1982). *Myofascial Pain and Dysfunction.* Baltimore: Williams and Wilkins.
7. Mennell J. M., Zohn D. A. (1976). *Musculoskeletal Pain.* Boston: Little, Brown.
8. Chrisman O. D., Mittnacht A., Snook G. A. (1964). A study of the results following rotatory manipulation in the lumbar intervertebral disc syndrome. *J. Bone Jt Surg;* **46A**:517–524.
9. Simons D. J., Day E., Goodell H., Wolff H. G. (1943). Experimental studies on headache. *Res. Publ. Ass. Nerv. Ment. Dis;* **23**:228–244.
10. Kleynhans A. M. (1980). Complications of and contraindications to spinal manipulative therapy. In *Modern Developments in the Principles and Practice of Chiropractic* (Haldeman S., ed.), pp. 359–389. East Norwall, Connecticut: Appleton–Century–Crofts.
11. Tissington Tatlow W. F., Bammer H. G. (1957). Syndrome of vertebral artery compression. *Neurology;* **7**:331–340.
12. Brown B. St J., Tissington Tatlow W. F. (1963). Radiographic studies of the vertebral arteries in cadavers. *Radiology;* **81**:80–88.
13. Maigne R. (1968). *Douleurs d'Origine Vertebrale et Traitements par Manipulations,* p. 144. Paris: Expansion Scientifique.
14. Sheehan S., Bauer R. B., Meyer J. S. (1960). Vertebral artery compression in cervical spondylosis. *J. Neurol;* **10**:968–986.
15. Greenman P. E. (1979). Lift therapy: use and abuse. *J.A.O.A;* **79**:238–250.

Chapter 13

What is the Cause of the Pain?

The precise nature of the changes which take place in an intervertebral joint which cause it to give rise to symptoms are still the subject of argument and of many conflicting theories. Nor is it known for certain why these symptoms, once started, so often tend to be recurrent, in spite of treatment. As has been stated earlier, there appears to be one certainty, namely that there is no 'little bone out of place'. With the exception of a small number of specific instances, also mentioned earlier, there is no subluxation, and certainly no dislocation, to be reduced.

There are relatively few basic physical signs which can be elicited in a sufficient proportion of back pain patients to justify the belief that they are fundamental to the condition. Two objective signs are almost always present, and indeed, if one looks in the right places, it is probably true to say that they are always present. These are loss of mobility and localised changes in tissue tension and texture. The diagnostic loss of mobility is that in the individual joint. There is one useful subjective sign. This is the tenderness which is found, unexpected by the patient, when one palpates an area of tissue change at a level of which the patient is not complaining. For example, many patients with a complaint of low back pain will have palpable dysfunction in the thoracolumbar region, as well as anything they may have lower down. When these areas of tissue change are palpated the patient will often exclaim, in some surprise, that the place is tender. If the tenderness is both localised and unexpected, it can be a valuable sign.

LOCALISED LOSS OF MOBILITY

In the acute phase, the loss of mobility is widespread but, when this is over, there remains a stiffness localised to one or more individual spinal joints or maybe to a part of the pelvic mechanism. There may be little or no loss of overall motion because it has been shown[1] that in the presence of a stiff spinal joint, the neighbouring joints develop an increased range. If more than one level becomes stiff, there will usually be some overall loss of range. This stiffness can be demonstrated both clinically and radiologically but both require special techniques, which have been described earlier (see Chapters 3, 4 and 5).

It is important that we should recognise that it is not necessarily correct to perform only an overall examination and to deduce from that that the mobility of that section of the spine is normal. Unfortunately, this still tends to happen and to lead to incorrect opinions being given in some legal and compensation cases.

Localised hypertonus

In the acute phase the muscle spasm is very obvious and no one will deny its existence. In the more chronic patient, careful examination may be required in order that localised tension abnormalities are not overlooked. Obesity makes it more difficult to detect subtle abnormalities of tissue tension and texture, but some people have a type of subcutaneous tissue through which it is quite difficult to feel. They are usually only moderately obese but the subcutaneous layer feels dense, as if it were more fibrous than normal. There does not appear to be any easy answer to examining that type of patient. They are disheartening, especially to the beginner in this field, but fortunately there are many more in whom palpation is relatively easy.

MULTIPLICITY OF LEVELS

Examination of the spine in patients who have a long history of back problems will usually reveal a number of levels where there is restricted motion. In these patients it may be difficult, at first, to find out which of the joints is the most important and it may not always be wise to try to treat all the levels at one session. It is common to find that at the first visit there are one or two levels where the tissue changes are well marked. The natural reaction is to treat those levels and it is usually best to do so. If these are the primary causes of the patient's back problem one can expect relief which may be well marked and lasting. If, however, the joints which one first finds are secondary, it may be that the improvement following treatment will be less good and relatively short lived. At the next examination it will be possible to find the more important levels rather more easily. It is likely that the levels treated originally will feel less abnormal and will not mask the tissue changes at the others. Sometimes treatment of secondary joints will actually aggravate the pain. This will also tend to happen if one has mistaken the level and treated the wrong joint. If the error was merely that of treating a secondary joint, there is likely to be some change for the better, often in mobility, even when the pain has been aggravated.

In patients who have a long history of symptoms it may be that one will find joints which were damaged long before and which have been accommodated for to the extent that they are no longer a significant part of the symptom-producing complex. It is not always easy at first to decide whether treatment should be given to a joint or not. The best guide is the presence of tissue tension and texture changes. It is important to define at what levels there is restriction of movement and asymmetry of position, but the decision as to whether to treat or not will depend more on the soft tissue changes. These changes may well alter during treatment of other levels so that it becomes clear that apparently silent levels do need to be treated after all. It is easy to give the advice that any positional abnormality should be treated, but sometimes this can be of more benefit to the manipulator's pocket book than to the patient's comfort!

THE HYPERMOBILE JOINT

The experimental evidence that stiffness at one spinal joint is usually

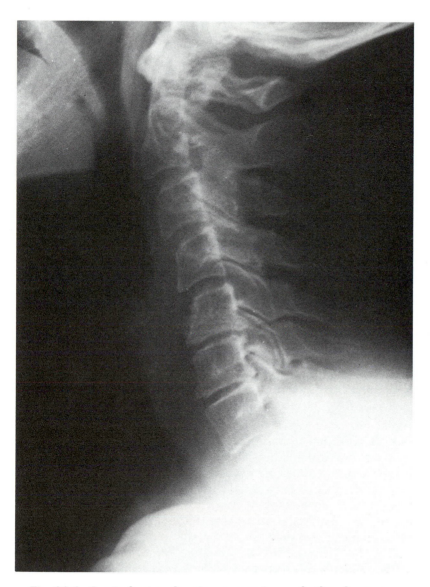

Fig. 13.1 Cervical spine showing narrowing and other degenerative changes at the C5–6 and C6–7 levels. Note the excessive forward projection of C4 on C5. In this case it is probably due to wearing away of the upper aspect of C5 by the movement occurring at the C4–5 level. This joint should be treated with caution and the appearance is a contraindication to high velocity treatment in that part of the neck.

accompanied by an increased range of motion in a neighbouring joint or joints has already been mentioned. In some patients one can find joints that are frankly hypermobile and this is a contraindication to high velocity manipulation at that joint. The evidence suggests that hypermobility is a reaction to treatable loss of mobility at another level. It is a mistake to feel that any manipulation is contraindicated because there happens to be a hypermobile joint nearby. The authors do not feel that sclerosant therapy is a good approach to this hypermobility, preferring to try to find the cause and treat, even, if necessary, by high velocity manipulation.

Hypermobility can sometimes be inferred from single position x-rays. Figure 13.1 is an example. There is narrowing and spur formation (especially posteriorly) at both the C5–6 and C6–7 disc levels. These joints will show restricted motion. At the C4–5 level there is some forward flexion of C4 which has caused loss of the usual lordosis, and there is also the appearance of erosion of the anterior aspect of the body of C5, suggesting that the C4–5 joint has been flexing further than is normal. This appearance is a contraindication to high velocity manipulation at that level, even if C4–5 seems to be the source of the symptoms. Muscle energy treatment can be given to neighbouring levels or even high velocity treatment rather further away. It is worth noting that, in many such patients, treatment of the dysfunctions in the upper thoracic spine will relieve the symptoms that appear to arise from the neck.

THE INTERVERTEBRAL DISC, VILLAIN OR ONLY COMPLICATION?

The paucity of clinical signs and the diversity of symptoms that can be produced by spinal joint disorders confused the medical profession to such an extent that they were not always recognised as being spinal in origin. The work of Mixter and Barr[2] stimulated interest in the intervertebral disc as a cause of symptoms. Since that time an immense amount of work has been done, but it appears that many of the pieces of the puzzle are still missing. There can be no doubt that actual protrusion and extrusion of disc material occurs and can cause physical pressure on nerve roots or on the cord itself. Such protrusion or extrusion in fact produces a space-occupying lesion in the spinal canal and may have to be distinguished from other such lesions. Even in this connection, however, there are a number of factors that require explanation.

First is the well established, but often forgotten, fact that pressure on nerve causes paralysis but no pain. An excellent example of this in the practice of one of the authors was a young man who had been sailing. He leaned against the side of the dinghy to balance the boat on a long reach lasting for more than half an hour. When he moved he found that he had a complete wrist drop with sensory as well as motor changes. The pressure on the radial nerve had been sufficient that it took more than 8 weeks to recover. He insisted that at no time did he have any pain.

The dural sleeve of the spinal nerve root is sensitive to certain types of stimulus. The anterior aspect of the dura is particularly sensitive and the nociceptor endings can be stimulated mechanically or chemically.[3] It appears, however, that the pain produced would be in the back, not in the leg.

Secondly, there is the occasional patient with unequivocal signs of disc protrusion with loss of motion and altered nerve conduction but no or almost no pain. These patients have had pain and are not of the unfortunate class of those with congenital absence of pain sensation.

Thirdly, there is the observation that, in many cases, symptoms of back and referred pain have been present for a long time before there is any evidence of an actual disc protrusion. When a true protrusion is found, a careful evaluation of the history will often fail to reveal any dramatic change in symptoms until there is sufficient pressure on the nerve to produce the different signs of a space-occupying lesion.

Charnley[4] was clearly unsatisfied that the disc was the primary cause of symptoms when he wrote:

> One of the most surprising things about acute lumbago is that the amount of pain does not seem to be proportional to the amount of organic change within the disc . . . We rarely find convincing protrusions in these cases but what is cogent to the present argument is that the material removed appeared more often to be normal than fibrous and stringy.

Friberg and Hult[5] found symptoms of sciatica in patients who did not have detectable herniation of discs, and Pedersen *et al.*[6] considered that they had evidence that back pain and sciatica could arise from stimulation of sinuvertebral nerve fibres.

There have been many who have thought that actual pressure from disc material was the main cause of the pain. Cyriax[7] maintained that he reduced protruded discs by his manipulations; Armstrong[8] actually gives diagrams of how a manipulation might move a nuclear sequestrum but goes on to condemn manipulation in any form. The older medical manipulators referred to the lesions as a fixation or strain without specifying a cause.

Anyone with experience in disc surgery will know that the nuclear material in a disc protrusion is not normal. Instead of being a firm, rubbery substance, it is composed of a softened sticky material which is somewhat stringy in consistency. From the anatomy of the disc we know that protrusion cannot take place until the nucleus is softened and a tear is made in the annulus through which the nuclear material can be forced. Except in the most superficial layers of the annulus, the intervertebral disc has no blood supply. It does not seem possible that an avascular tissue could heal, almost instantly, a track through which a nucleus had protruded, even if reduction were possible.

If one tries hard enough, it is possible to suck back excess toothpaste into the tube; if then you tread on the tube with the top off, it all comes out again. Nachemson and Morris[9] recorded the pressure inside intervertebral discs in various positions. Their figures vary from a minimum of 50 kg/cm² standing, to a maximum of 100–127 kg/cm² when seated.

This pressure would surely cause softened material to protrude again if there were a preformed track down which it could go.

These theoretical considerations suggest that continuous traction would be more likely to be effective in both securing and maintaining reduction. In practice it does not seem to happen that way. Traction is sometimes of value in treatment, especially of those with very acute pain and spasm, but the authors know of no recorded instances of successful reduction of disc protrusions by this means.

SYMPTOMS FROM JOINTS THAT HAVE NO INTERVERTEBRAL DISC

As was pointed out earlier, there are two joints in the spine that have no intervertebral discs, but which can still be the source of symptoms strictly comparable to those seen in joint lesions in other parts of the spine. Reference has also been made to the fact that similar symptoms can arise from dysfunction of the sacroiliac joint.

The concept that the sacroiliac joint could be the cause of symptoms was put forward in 1911 by Goldthwaite[10] and again in 1938 by Gray.[11] Both authors recorded instances of dramatic relief following manipulation of the sacroiliac joint. In spite of this, the medical profession has commonly exhibited blank disbelief (once shared by at least one of the authors!) at the idea that the sacroiliac joint could be the cause of symptoms and, more particularly, of referred symptoms. This disbelief almost certainly stems from the teaching of the medical schools and the not unnatural blind acceptance of this teaching by the student. The attitude of the teachers appears to have resulted from the medical profession's preoccupation with the intervertebral disc as the cause of the trouble, and the belief that for the production of referred pain, actual pressure on nerves or nerve roots was required. There is, of course, no nerve of any size on which pressure can conceivably be brought by a minor movement of the sacroiliac joint.

Three specific instances of relief of pain from manipulation of the sacroiliac joint from the practice of one of the authors follow.

1. **Pain in the low back**. A 34-year-old female presented with a 4-year history of intermittent back pain. There had been a further acute attack 2 weeks before. She had had a below-knee amputation of the right leg 10 years previously. Examination showed that, when standing, the right side of the pelvis was significantly higher than the left and the dysfunction was localised to the right sacroiliac joint. Measurement of the difference in leg length by the x-ray technique showed that the limb was more than 2.5 cm (1 inch) too long. Treatment of the sacroiliac joint on a total of seven occasions resulted in marked relief. The limb was also adjusted.

2. **Pain referred to the heel**. A girl aged 7 gave a history of having jumped from a roof 2.4 metres (8 feet) high, about 10 days before. She complained of being unable to bear weight on her left heel. Examination

did not show any abnormality in the heel and x-rays were normal. Examination of the low back showed a sacroiliac strain which required two treatments by manipulation to give complete relief. There had been no back pain and no pain in the leg except at the heel.

3. **Pain referred to the knee.** A girl aged 13 complained of pain in the front of the knee and said that she had fallen on it 2 weeks before. The only abnormality in the knee was a very tender prepatellar nodule, but examination of the low back did show a sacroiliac strain. There was no history of previous back trouble and she did not admit to having any back discomfort. One treatment of the sacroiliac joint by manipulation stopped the pain but she attended once more, 2 months later, for a recurrence caused by a further fall.

THE EVIDENCE FROM THE EFFECTS OF LOCAL ANAESTHETIC INJECTION

Injections of local anaesthetic can relieve pain in a way that makes it clear that it is not, in those cases, due to some change in the disc itself, with or without the production of nerve or nerve root pressure.

Occasionally a patient is seen with acutely tender areas in peripheral muscle, whether they are true trigger points or the more generalised condition which has been called fibrositis in Chapter 12. In some of these patients, injection of the tender areas may result in dramatic relief not only of the local symptoms but also of both the referred pain and the back pain. In those in whom the relief is not that dramatic or long lasting, there may be enough change in the symptoms to show that the peripheral muscle is acting as a secondary focus for the production of symptoms. It is probable that the symptoms are often started by a spinal joint dysfunction. Such a joint dysfunction may also be the cause of the changes in the peripheral muscle which later can maintain the symptoms, even when the spinal joint has settled.

In an occasional patient, the caudal epidural injection of a weak solution of local anaesthetic will relieve both the local and the referred pain before there is any evidence of change in either sensory or motor function in the low lumbar nerves. This suggests that the mechanism involves the sinuvertebral nerves or the plexus of nerves that surrounds the paravertebral venous system, or even the articular and periosteal branches of the posterior primary division of the spinal nerve roots, all of which have fibres with thin myelin sheaths. The fibres in the spinal nerve roots are less easily accessible to the solution and most have thicker myelin sheaths and would be affected less easily.

That the disc must play some part in the production of symptoms is shown by work done by Lindblom[12] and Perey.[13] They showed that when a needle is introduced into a disc in order to perform a discogram, the posterior longitudinal ligament is sensitive. The pain was only severe if the disc was abormal. When the needle advanced into the nucleus no pain was felt. When the solution was injected into a normal disc it produced a mild pain in the low back. In a disc which was abnormal, but not ruptured, both the back pain and the sciatica were reproduced. This happened even when the solution contained 1% of novocaine, which suggests that the effect was in some way connected with pressure on surrounding structures rather than anything in the disc itself.

The importance of the true disc protrusion must not be overlooked. The dramatic relief which can follow surgical removal of a large disc protrusion is most gratifying to both patient and surgeon. Unfortunately, surgery for back pain with or without referred pain is not always so satisfying, and cases that are initially successful will sometimes have further acute recurrences or may develop less acute symptoms that can be enough to prevent the patient doing certain types of work. A typical case of acute recurrence in the practice of one of the authors was a bank manager who had had very successful surgery for a disc protrusion 7 years before. The pain had begun to return 1 week before he was seen. It had come on without known cause and had quickly become severe. When seen, no abnormal neurological signs were found, although straight leg raising was much reduced. He responded very well to treatment by manipulation and became pain free in about five treatments. The pain was described as being the same as before his surgery and this is probably an example of a pain referred from a different structure but felt in the same place as in the previous episode.

The changes in the intervertebral disc in those who have actual protrusions are accepted as being due to degeneration. The cause of the degeneration has not been agreed but it is assumed by many to be due to trauma. Roaf[14] said: 'Prolapse of a normal disc either never or hardly ever occurs. It is only when the nucleus pulposus has lost its normal characteristics—probably through poor nutrition subsequent to ischaemia, secondary to infection or trauma—that prolapse of the disc material takes place.'

Major protrusions of disc material requiring surgery for their relief are uncommon in the young but by no means unheard of. The youngest known to the authors was a girl of 11. She had signs of a space-occupying lesion which proved at surgery to be a large protrusion and she made an excellent recovery after the surgery. It is difficult to believe that a child of 11 could be suffering from idiopathic degeneration of her discs. Could it be due to loss of mobility at that joint?

THE MECHANISM OF DISC NUTRITION

It is well known that there are no blood vessels in the intervertebral disc except in the most superficial layers of the annulus. There is no suggestion, however, that the material is not alive. The most accurate descriptions of normal nuclear material suggest that it is made of mesenchymal cells in a three-dimensional lattice-work of fine collagen fibres covered with mucopolysaccharides and containing a high proportion of water.[15] As in any other part of the body, the living cells must be supplied with nourishment and must have their waste products removed in order to remain alive. The mechanism of nutrition of the disc is said to be by a colloid imbibition pump.[15,16] Colloid substances have the property of attracting fluid. This property is known as the imbibition pressure. In the intervertebral disc, this tendency is balanced by the action of the hydraulic pressure which has the effect of trying to squeeze out fluid from the disc substance. When the disc imbibes fluid, its size increases, the fibres in the fibrocartilaginous annulus become taut and, even if there were neither superincumbent weight nor muscle action, the imbibition process would reach a point of equilibrium. This is because of the hydrostatic pressure exerted on the disc substance by the end-plates of the vertebral bodies above and below, and the fibrocartilage of the annulus around the sides. That the process of imbibition can continue is shown by the fact that when a horizontal section is made through a normal disc and the cut surface is then immersed in saline, the nuclear material swells and rises above the level of the surrounding annulus. When the patient sits down or bends forwards, the hydrostatic pressure increases on the disc nucleus [9] and it is probable that this increased pressure squeezes fluid out through the foramina in the vertebral end-plate into the cancellous bone of the vertebral body. The rich blood supply of this bone is well equipped to remove metabolites and supply nutrients to the tissue fluid. When the posture is changed to one in which the hydraulic pressure is lower, a fresh supply of fluid containing nutrients is sucked back by the imbibition pressure into the disc.

If this is a correct explanation of the process of disc nutrition, it is but a small step to assume that this imbibition pump is dependent for its function on the mobility of the intervertebral joint at that level. When one considers the structure of the intervertebral joint as a whole and the pressure to which it is subjected, it is probably unreasonable to say that the loss of movement would, except rarely, be so complete as to prevent the pump working at all. On the other hand, it seems certain that the efficiency of such a pump would be interfered with by stiffness such that no movement is detectable on x-ray examination in flexion and extension. That there can be this degree of loss of mobility in spinal joint injuries is established.

Thus it can be argued that the intervertebral joint stiffness secondary to injury may cause defective nutrition of the disc. It is tempting to think that the observed nuclear degeneration in actual disc protrusions is due to this defect in nutrition. The suggestion that the loss of nutrition is partial rather than absolute could be part of the explanation of the delay, so often observed, between the original injury and the appearance of any sign of a true disc protrusion.

THE NEUROLOGICAL EVIDENCE

Wyke[3,17] has shown that there are three routes by which pain fibres reach the dorsal root ganglion from the spinal canal: the sinuvertebral nerves, the plexus around the paravertebral venous system and branches of the posterior rami which supply the apophyseal joints, the periosteum and the related fasciae of the surfaces of the vertebral bodies and their arches, the interspinous ligaments and the blood vessels.

According to Wyke, the receptor endings of these nerves (and the nerves themselves) can only be caused to discharge by either mechanical or chemical irritation. Mechanical causes can be:

1. abnormal postural stress;
2. local oedema, from either direct trauma or acute inflammation;
3. direct compression;
4. excessive distension of veins in the paravertebral plexus.

Chemical irritants may be:

1. irritants associated with inflammation or with sustained muscle activity;
2. much less commonly, iatrogenic (contrast media etc.).

Stimulation of these pain receptor systems causes reflex contraction of related muscles which, if sustained, can itself give rise to chemical irritation of the receptor endings, closing the circle. In this way Wyke says that *muscular pain may become superimposed on and actually become more important than the primary spinal pain*. He also points out that the reflex spasm produced by a visceral lesion can cause a spinal pain-spasm-pain cycle which is self-perpetuating.

Wyke makes many interesting observations, some of which are opposed to classical neuroanatomical teaching. Nociceptor afferent innervation of dermatomes is not unisegmental. The sinuvertebral nerves have branches that extend over at least four segments, and the innervation in the lumbar region is by branches from between three and five dorsal nerve roots. No joint in the lumbosacral region has monosegmental innervation, and from this he deduces that denervation by transcutaneous procedures is not possible. He also says: 'Contrary to the traditional opinions of many doctors, inflammatory disorders of the back muscles and their related connective tissues are seldom the cause of back pain except as a complication of some acute febrile illness.'

EXPERIMENTAL WORK ON THE SUBJECT OF REFERRED PAIN

The problem of referred pain is one which has received much attention from neurologists, anatomists and physiologists. Kellgren[18] reports work started by Lewis and carried on by himself in which an irritant solution of 6% saline was injected into volunteers at various sites. He showed that by injecting the irritant beside the spinous process of the 1st sacral vertebra, he could produce the typical pain of sciatica with radiation all down the leg. The manner in which the injection was given makes it likely that, in addition to the muscle, the saline would have affected ligaments and possibly the periosteum on the back of the lamina of the 1st sacral vertebra. A similar injection at the 1st lumbar level produced a typical attack of lumbago. Similar experiments have been done by others[19,20,21] and a discussion of this work is given by Troup.[22] Many of the workers in this field have noted that referred pain is associated with hyperalgesia in the area to which the pain is referred and this is commonly accompanied by cutaneous hypoaesthesia in the same area. The suggestion has been made that there is both a distal and a central mechanism involved in the production of referred pain, and that the central mechanism probably involves both the spinal cord and higher centres.

It appears that it is not necessary to have actual damage to the segmental nerve root in order to have referred pain. What is more, it has been shown that the experimental referred pain from these injections is not necessarily confined to the dermatome, myotome or sclerotome of that level.[21]

Inflammation

The evidence for inflammation as a cause of pain in the spine is largely based on the therapeutic results of measures designed to reduce any inflammatory reaction. It is interesting to speculate on the cause of this reaction. Wyke's work suggests that it may be mechanical but also that it could be chemical, resulting from continuing hypertonus in muscle. For the present, empirical diagnosis and treatment appear to be appropriate.

IS TIGHT MUSCLE THE MAIN CAUSE OF PAIN?

The theory that, in spinal joint derangements, the immediate cause of pain is the tight muscle is an attractive one in many ways. There must be very few people who have never experienced muscle pain from cramp. The chemical irritation of muscle by hypertonic saline is known to produce referred pain. One of the most significant common factors in the wide variety of available treatments appears to be their ability to promote relaxation in muscle. That peripheral muscles can cause specific patterns of referred pain has been demonstrated clearly by Travell, Mennell, Simons and others in publications previously referred to. They have also shown that, if the abnormally tight portion of the muscle is made to relax, the pain goes. It has also been shown that irritation of deep muscles, and other mesodermal tissue, around the spinal joint will cause referred pain similar to clinical syndromes.[18–21,23,24]

Korr[25] gives experimental evidence for the existence of spindle dysfunction with overaction of the gamma system in the dysfunctional muscles. The concept of a muscle in which the resting length adjustment has been 'turned up' to near the maximum tightness appears to fit with clinical observations. The joint stiffness is rarely absolute. Movement away from the painful direction is nearly always possible but there remains a barrier to movement, particularly in one direction. It seems reasonable to argue that this is what would happen if the muscles on one aspect of the joint were abnormally tight.

The precise means by which the sensation of pain is produced is not clear. It is tempting to blame it on accumulation of pain-producing metabolites resulting from the overactivity which keeps the muscle tight. On the other hand, it is difficult to see how the circulation in the muscle could be significantly compromised by the degree of tightness required to produce even the maximum shortening of its resting length. It may be that the explanation will be found to be, in part at least, an overflow of the continuing afferent discharge in the gamma system. Wyke's work, referred to above, did cause him to favour the metabolite explanation.

REFERENCES

1. Froning E. C., Frohman B. (1968). Motion of the lumbar spine after laminectomy and spine fusion. *J. Bone Jt Surg;* 50:879–918.
2. Mixter W. J., Barr J. S. (1934). Rupture of the intervertebral disc with involvement of the spinal canal. *New Engl. J. Med;* 211:210–215.
3. Wyke B. (1970). The neurological basis of spinal pain. *Rheumatol. Phys. Med;* 10:356–366.
4. Charnley J. (1958). Physical change in the prolapsed disc. *Lancet;* 2:43–44.
5. Friberg S., Hult L. (1951). Comparative study of abrodil myelogram and operative findings. *Acta orthop. Scand;* 20:303–314.
6. Pedersen H. E., Blunk C. F. J., Gardner E. (1956). Anatomy of the lumbo-sacral posterior rami. *J. Bone Jt Surg;* 38A:377–391.
7. Cyriax J. (1955). *Textbook of Orthopaedic Medicine*, 5th edn. London: Cassell.
8. Armstrong J. R. (1965). *Lumbar Disc Lesions*, 3rd edn. London: Livingstone.
9. Nachemson A., Morris J. H. (1964). In vivo measurements of intradiscal pressure. *J. Bone Jt Surg;* 46A:1077–1092.
10. Goldthwaite G. (1911). The lumbo–sacral articulation. *Boston Med. Surg. J;* 164:365–372.
11. Gray H. (1938). Sacro-iliac joint pain. *Int. Clin;* 2:54–96.
12. Lindblom K. (1951). Technique and results of diagnostic disc puncture and injection. *Acta orthopaed. Scand;* 20:315–326.
13. Perey O. (1951). Contrast medium examination of the intervertebral discs. *Acta orthopaed. Scand;* 20:327–334.
14. Roaf R. (1958). Physical changes in the prolapsed disc. *Lancet;* 2:265–266.
15. Hendry N. G. C. (1958). The hydration of the nucleus pulposus. *J. Bone Jt Surg;* 40B:132–144.
16. Sylven B. (1951). On the biology of the nucleus pulposus. *Acta orthopaed. Scand;* 20:275–279.
17. Wyke B. (1980). The neurology of low back pain. In *The Lumbar Spine and Back Pain*, 2nd edn. (Jayson M., ed.) pp. 265–339. Tunbridge Wells: Pitman Medical.
18. Kellgren J. H. (1949). Deep pain sensibility. *Lancet;* 1:943–949.
19. Sinclair D. C., Feindel W. H., Weddell G., Falconer M. A. (1948). The intervertebral ligaments as a source of referred pain. *J. Bone Jt Surg;* 30B:514–521.
20. Feinstein C., Langlin J. N. K., Jameson R. M., Schiller F. (1954). Experiments in pain referred from deep somatic structures. *J. Bone Jt Surg;* 36A:981–997.
21. Hockaday J. M., Whitty C. W. M. (1967). Patterns of referred pain in normal subjects. *Brain;* 90:481–496.

22. Troup J. D. G. (1968). PhD thesis, London University.
23. Kellgren J. H. (1939). On the distribution of pain arising from deep somatic structures. *Clin. Sci;* 4:35–46.
24. Lewis T., Kellgren J. H. (1939). Observations relating to referred pain. *Clin. Sci;* 4:47–71.
25. Korr I. M. (1975). Proprioceptors and somatic dysfunction. *J.A.O.A;* 74:638–650.

Chapter 14

Clinical Observations

Low back pain permeates society with profound economic implications. The statistics contradict the study that claims that 70–90% of low back sufferers will be well within 3 months.[1] It may be true to say that the acute symptoms will have abated within 3 months, but the patients are not likely to be well. People with joint dysfunction who are engaged in physical labour are apt to suffer recurrence of symptoms on return to work. Those with occupations that are less demanding physically may manage reasonably well and believe themselves to have recovered. The common statement that they have to be 'careful' of their back implies less than full recovery. It is absurd to find otherwise healthy workmen shelved with pensions for their back injury when all they have is a simple and reversible problem.

It has sometimes been noted with surprise that people who are familiar with manipulation consider it an 'alternative', more desirable than surgery because it is not invasive. The fact is that the alternative is in the diagnosis, the conditions discussed in this book are not surgical problems. Joint dysfunction is not amenable to surgery, nor are surgical conditions, such as a major extrusion of disc material, amenable to treatment by manipulation. Manipulation, in the wide sense of the word, is the treatment for joint dysfunction in the musculoskeletal system when that is present.

In this connection it is worth pointing out that it is impossible to perform a laminectomy without doing a manipulation of the lower back. This may account for some of the good results that follow surgery even when the exploration was negative for disc protrusion or other pathology. The effect of such 'manipulation' seems a more likely reason for improvement than anything to do with the so-called bulging disc to which symptoms are often ascribed.

TRANSITIONAL AREAS

The transitional areas of the spine seem to have a propensity for dysfunction. The occipitoatlantal articulation, the cervicothoracic junction, the thoracolumbar junction and the lumbosacral junction are key areas which are responsible for a variety of pain syndromes. Some of these can be the subject of extensive and expensive investigation if the physician is unaware of or unskilled in methods of manual examination. The symptoms often have their immediate cause in other more obvious lesions, and without careful screening of the transitional areas, joint restriction at these junctions may escape notice. If so, the relief from dealing with the symptomatic area is likely to be brief and the patient will return, often complaining of an altered pattern of pain distribution or of a totally different set of symptoms. One would presume that the transitional areas are particularly vulnerable to force, or to unguarded movement or to prolonged maintenance of one position because of the stress produced by the change at these junctions from greater to less mobility. The key vertebra is not necessarily the one at the expected level and, as pointed out in Chapter 2, the functional change is not always at the same level. This is especially true at the thoracolumbar junction.

In emphasising the junctional areas, the intention is to stress the frequency of their involvement and the ease with which problems there can be overlooked. It is not to imply that screening of other parts of the spine is unimportant.

The occipitoatlantal articulation

This seems invariably to be involved in neck injuries such as whiplash. The pattern of cephalgia seems to be typical of an upper cervical lesion: patients complaining of recurrent occipital headaches radiating from the neck up, travelling anteriorly and often settling retro-orbitally on one or both sides. Complaints of visual disturbances are common, taking the form of difficulty in focusing or blurring of vision. Ophthalmological investigation usually fails to detect any actual visual abnormality. A complaint of dizziness, not necessarily vertigo, is a common feature and sometimes there is nausea also. The patient may be labelled as suffering from the 'post-concussion syndrome' and later may be considered to have atypical migraine, although a preheadache aura is not usually a feature.

Recurrent cephalgia after trauma may have its primary basis in 'blockage' in the upper cervical spine, but the cranial bones are almost invariably implicated. This controversial subject will not be discussed here, but interested readers are advised to consult works on osteopathic craniosacral theory.[2,3] It is appropriate to acknowledge that headache is a non-specific symptom and often has other causes in addition to or instead of structural dysfunction of the musculoskeletal system.

Great care must be exercised in treating lesions of the upper cervical spine, in particular the occipitoatlantal joint. The path of the vertebral arteries as they enter the cranial cavity through the foramen magnum makes them particularly vulnerable to force at this level of the spine. Evidence of occlusion of one of the vertebral arteries when the neck is fully rotated and extended has been well documented. The risk of vasospasm after forceful manoeuvres in the upper cervical spine, with potentially catastrophic consequences, has already been discussed in Chapter 12. To position a neck in extension and full rotation is unwise, it is considered to be safer to maintain some degree of flexion. Only muscle energy (or isometric) or indirect techniques are recommended and this book no longer gives a description of a thrusting technique for this joint. It is appreciated, however, that much manipulation, and indeed what most people associate with the idea of manipulation, is of the direct thrust type and is used frequently in the neck. It is fair to say that the incidence of complications is very low but the consequences can be so serious that it is essential to avoid any unnecessary risk. It is clear that the potential for a vascular accident can be minimised by careful localisation of the barrier and by cautious and gentle management.

The pain threshold of the individual determines the tolerance to constantly recurring pain syndromes, but cephalgia secondary to cervical lesions appears to be particularly devastating. A patient of one of the authors would not accept a promotion in a sports organisation because he knew that he would not succeed because of recurrent disabling headaches. There are many examples of patients who found that returning to work was intolerable in similar circumstances. These individuals are often considered to be suffering from stress or psychological factors and, indeed, recurrent occipital pain does have psychological implications. The treatment, however, is not counselling!

The cervicothoracic junction

This is another common area responsible for marked pain which can be confused at times with a root syndrome, or with bursitis in the shoulder, or a thoracic outlet syndrome, or a disc herniation. Pain radiating down the arm to the hand suggests radicular involvement, and the paraesthesiae influenced by posture or movement confirm the impression. Radiological evidence of disc narrowing at the C5–6 vertebral level sometimes leads to surgical intervention such as Cloward's procedure, particularly when the symptoms are severe and physical measures such as traction fail to provide relief.

Manual examination in fact may determine that there is dysfunction at the C5–6 vertebral level but it is more likely that it is lower, probably in the upper thoracic spine, and blockage at the T1 vertebral level is much more common. It is helpful if tenderness is found in the adjacent tissues, but localised pain is not always present. The upper thoracic spine is a more difficult area to diagnose because normal movement is much less than in other areas of the spine and detection of restriction depends on very subtle findings. This area of the spine has profound importance with widespread manifestations. Sympathetic dystrophy is discussed later under contusions and fractures but its cause is likely to be found in this area of the spine. There can be marked effects on the autonomic system and inferences or claims by manipulators of various kinds that this treatment has effects on various organs, including cardiac muscle, probably has its basis in this fact.

Carpal tunnel syndromes, ulnar entrapment neuropathies, and lateral epicondylitis are not always straightforward localised lesions, as one might think, even in the presence of mild changes in nerve conduction. In such patients it is always wise to screen the upper thoracic spine for mechanical problems.

Chest wall pain can often be traced to this area of the spine and costochondritis is an interesting secondary manifestation of thoracic joint dysfunction. If the thoracic spinal dysfunction is treated, the costochondritis will usually settle within a short time.

The thoracolumbar junction

The thoracolumbar syndrome has been discussed at length by Robert Maigne.[4] This area can be the site of origin of low back pain and is very often involved as a secondary dysfunction in those who have had primary problems in the lower joints for any length of time. Diffuse pain syndromes of variable distribution are often found to originate here. Localised tenderness is not always present, and careful screening of this area may be rewarding, particularly when sacroiliac or lower lumbar lesions have been found. Failure to deal with this problem is likely to result in an unsatisfactory outcome to treatment of the more obvious problems. In spite of its importance, this area may be almost silent on localised examination.

The lumbosacral junction

A lumbosacral lesion can be found as a single entity, but is usually a component of sacroiliac dysfunction. It is hard at times to decide whether the L5 facet is actually restricted in movement, or whether the position of the vertebra simply reflects the influence of the orientation of the sacrum, when there is a concurrent sacroiliac lesion. In cases where there is both a lumbar facet syndrome and a sacroiliac lesion, it is recommended that the lumbar spine is treated first in order to avoid exacerbating the pain. This is more likely to happen if the lumbar lesion is maladaptive to the pelvic dysfunction.

SACROILIAC JOINTS

Despite more than 50 years of documentation to the contrary, some physicians still consider that the sacroiliac joints do not move. These joints are complex and not fully understood, but it is clear to the authors that they can have a profound effect on body mechanics. The argument regarding movement was discussed at length in Chapter 2 and will not be re-opened here, except to say that anyone who still holds the view that these joints are immobile can never hope to achieve control of common back pain.

The sacroiliac joint appears to be the single greatest cause of back pain. The range of motion is small and difficult to describe but, when normal joint play is lost, agonising pain can be precipitated and this may be in the distribution of the sciatic nerve. It is clear that there cannot be actual pressure on the sciatic nerve from any simple dysfunction of the sacroiliac joint. The pattern of referred pain is variable, it may be in the buttock or the groin or even to the genitalia. It is often in the thigh but not so commonly below the knee. Pain on the lateral aspect of the greater trochanter is much more commonly due to sacroiliac (or lumbar) joint dysfunction than to bursitis. Pain in the hip region may be burning in character and suggest meralgia paraesthetica; there may even be restriction of hip joint motion.

The so-called pyriformis syndrome is usually due to dysfunction in the sacroiliac joint, but it must be recognised that the pyriformis is very often hypertonic in association with such a lesion and may well require stretching to regain its normal resting length. If this is neglected, the sacroiliac lesion is likely to recur rapidly.

It is reasonable to suggest that on confronting a patient in severe pain of sciatic distribution, the first thought should be 'sacroiliac' not 'disc', even if only because of the statistical probability. The differentiation of a mechanical joint lesion from a herniation of nucleus pulposus can be difficult if there is no frank neurological deficit. A sharp increase in lumbosacral pain on rapid dorsiflexion of the foot with the leg elevated suggests radicular pain but is not conclusive. Sacroiliac lesions can co-exist with disc herniations and an example of such a patient who returned rapidly to work after sacroiliac treatment is given in Chapter 12. In cases of doubt it is wise to restrict manipulation to muscle energy techniques, and fortunately these are usually very effective for the sacroiliac joints. A known disc herniation is not a contraindication to properly designed manipulative treatment and many patients respond in such a way that any question of surgical treatment is forgotten.

DEGENERATIVE DISC DISEASE

Even respected, knowledgeable physicians frequently ascribe back pain to 'degenerative disc disease'.[5] Radiological evidence of disc narrowing and changes compatible with degeneration appear first to become evident in the fourth decade and progress gradually with age. The progression is apparently inexorable but there is no evidence that this is a painful process. There is no study which shows any correlation between this radiological finding and the incidence of back pain.[6] It is likely that in this process the human spine loses some of its shock absorbing ability and may therefore be less able to withstand trauma. The rate of progress of the changes appears to be influenced by genetic factors and does depend in part on the stresses to which the individual subjects his spine. For example, weight lifters and those engaged in heavy labour tend to have accelerated degeneration. The lack of correlation between the radiological findings and the incidence of back pain still holds.

Patients presenting with back pain often have no radiological findings of significance except evidence of disc degeneration. It is perhaps not surprising that physicians who have no knowledge of the examination techniques of manual medicine will conclude that the degenerative changes are the cause. The idea that back pain is the inevitable result of ageing is not supported by the statistical evidence and certainly loses its credibility when one learns to examine for normal joint play and for joint blockage.

It is interesting to note that lumbar fusions for back pain are no longer regarded as good treatment in the opinion of many surgeons. The same is not true of cervical fusion, which is still often performed, especially at the C5–6 level. When this is based on nothing more than pain in the C5 nerve root distribution and radiological changes at that level, it often is, in the opinion of the authors, a sad misapplication of surgical skill.

ANATOMICAL VARIANTS

Spondylolisthesis

This is encountered periodically among low back pain patients. Statistics[6] suggest that there is no correlation between incidence of the defect and clinical low back pain. There is still some argument as to the cause of spondylolisthesis and the spondylolysis which is believed to be its precursor. There is clear evidence of a familial incidence but it does appear to be more common in those who expose their back to certain types of strain during their early years. The significance for treatment by manual medicine procedures depends on how stable the segment is. If the segment is unstable, or hypermobile, manipulation at that level is contraindicated. If there is major instability, and the more so if there is evidence of cauda equina pressure, surgery may be indicated.

Even when the segment is unstable, it is often not the source of the symptoms. In most patients with spondylolisthesis careful structural examination will show evidence of blockage at a different level, often several segments higher. It is always worth checking the low thoracic joints. There is no contraindication even to thrusting treatment at these joints, but it is important that the localisation is accurate and the more so if it is a joint close to the defective segment. There does not appear to be any contraindication to the use of a muscle energy procedure except at a joint that is grossly hypermobile.

Abnormal segmentation

Sacralisation, lumbarisation and joints between the lumbar transverse processes and the ilium are sometimes blamed for back pain. It is the authors' firm opinion that these are to be regarded as incidental radiographic findings indicating anatomical variants. There is no evidence that they are painful conditions and the finding should not be an excuse for failure to make a careful search for dysfunctional segments in the pelvis, the lumbar or even the thoracic spine.

Cervical ribs are also an anatomical variant and, although there is evidence that they can cause vascular problems, they are often an incidental finding of no clinical importance. Dysfunction of joints at the cervicothoracic junction and in the upper thoracic spine is very often the cause of symptoms that could be ascribed to abnormal ribs and it is wise therefore to exclude such problems (or to treat them!) before considering surgery.

Obesity

This is also generally considered as a factor in the generation of back pain. The overweight individual with pendulous abdomen certainly fits the concept of increased shear stress on the lumbar facets. This reasoning is not supported statistically and it has not been established that fat people suffer more from back pain than those of normal weight. It is convenient to blame gluttony but, in the experience of both the authors, those who do succeed in losing weight do not lose their back pain any better than those who do not take the trouble. There is no doubt that fat people are more difficult to handle. The adipose tissue makes diagnosis a lot less easy and the sheer bulk of some makes treatment difficult, even for a large man.

OSTEOARTHRITIS OF THE HIP

One of the most misleading situations can be encountered when the source of the pain seems obvious but the remedy is ineffective. This can happen in those with osteoarthritis of the hip. Even in the presence of considerable restriction of movement of the hip joint, it is wise to consider other causes of pain before concluding that the hip itself is totally or mainly responsible. Pain referred to the hip area is common from both sacroiliac and lumbar joint dysfunction and treatment of these is easier and much less expensive than either conservative or surgical treatment of the hip itself. Manual medicine treatment can sometimes be used as a diagnostic test. If correctly performed at a dysfunctional level, it will do no harm to the hip and can be continued in those for whom it proves helpful.

Total hip relacement can give dramatic relief of true hip pain, but examination of the lower spine and pelvis by the techniques of manual medicine is advisable before surgery because concomitant pelvic or lumbar dysfunction is almost universal. These dysfunctions are likely to be a significant cause of additional pain in many patients, possibly because of disturbances of spinal mechanics secondary to the restriction of hip motion.

Both authors have seen numerous patients for whom surgery gave partial relief only and there did not appear to be anything wrong with the procedure. Rather, there was clear evidence of dysfunction in the spine or pelvis, sometimes even as high as the thoracic spine.

CHEST WALL PAIN

Chest wall pain often results in a cardiac investigation. It has been estimated that 40% of cases presenting at emergency departments with symptoms indistinguishable from angina do not have myocardial ischaemia. Pain radiating across the trapezius muscle, down the arm and across the pectoral muscles is a common manifestation of upper thoracic joint dysfunction. Treatment of this problem is routine in a manual medicine practice. Screening of the upper thoracic spine should be part and parcel of an examination for cardiac involvement. Rapid relief of symptoms after mobilisation of an upper thoracic lesion is a pleasing outcome; expensive procedures such as stress testing and cardiac catheterisation are rendered unnecessary.

The differential diagnosis of angina, or of what seems to be angina, includes the investigation of possible sources of pain in the thoracic spine, and a finding of joint dysfunction can provide an easy explanation. This is acceptable when there is no evidence of cardiac impairment, but more controversial is the role of joint dysfunction in angina which is without doubt of cardiac origin. This concept is discussed later in the section on organic disease (see p. 237).

ABDOMINAL PAIN

The clinician is obliged to look for the most likely causes of pain in any examination, and the abdomen is no exception. Gastrointestinal causes, the liver, or renal disease are all usually considered carefully, but we have not been trained to think of another source which is referred pain from blockage of thoracic or lumbar spinal joints. It used to be held by accrediting bodies that a certain percentage of appendices removed for the 'acute abdomen' should be normal, because otherwise a number of cases of acute appendicitis would be missed, with serious consequences to the patient. While that kind of thinking may have its merits, there seems to have been no ensuing inquiry as to what the problem was when the appendix proved to be normal. As with any other pain, the cause can be spinal and, if it is, it can be discovered and dealt with rapidly before entering into serological or organic function tests, contrast studies, or exploratory laparotomy.

PREGNANCY

Pregnancy is often associated with back pain. The shifting of the centre of gravity as the uterus enlarges puts increasing stress on the lumbar spine. Such cases invariably display joint dysfunction; it is likely that the advancing pregnancy decompensates for previously quiescent joint restriction, or perhaps the increased stress precipitates such a problem. Regardless of whether or not the joint restriction was present before the pregnancy, manipulation can give immense relief. As the pregnancy advances it becomes increasingly difficult to make a diagnosis simply because of physical factors. It should still be possible to determine if the sacroiliac joints are involved, and motion testing can impart a sense of restriction elsewhere, depending on one's tactile skills. During the first 3 or 4 months there should not be any real problem in making a full diagnosis. Isometric or muscle energy techniques can be carried out without any real problem and do not expose the patient to premature labour. One of the authors has long experience of using thrusting techniques on pregnant patients but because of incomplete implantation he never did this at the time of the first three missed periods. He did not see a single complication of this treatment.

Some physiotherapy departments will refuse to treat pregnant patients because of the fear of litigation. This attitude may be wise in view of the widespread use of heat modalities with effects on the fetus that may not be fully known. On the other hand, there need not be any fear of using manual methods of articulation or muscle energy manipulation for those who have acquired the skills. The authors are unaware of any untoward effects on mother or fetus from such treatment and it can give great relief.

In some patients the back pain appears to start with delivery and the assumption that this results from straining may well be correct. In such cases, sacroiliac dysfunction is common but the symphysis pubis should not be forgotten, and that is one of the dysfunctions that can often be demonstrated radiologically.

CONTUSIONS AND FRACTURES

It is clear that trauma severe enough to result in fractures and contusions is also likely to have precipitated less severe injuries to the spine. Spinal joint dysfunction can be the source of symptoms in unexpected places. Adequate treatment of a wrist fracture, for example, does not obviate the necessity of searching for other sources of pain in those who do not settle as they should. The cervical and upper thoracic spine are often such an additional source. Head injuries are commonly complicated by dysfunction in cervical joints and symptoms such as post-concussion headache can often be markedly relieved if the spinal joints are treated. This is not in any way to suggest that the most pressing injury should not be treated first. It must be remembered that instability is a contraindication and that manipulation can be intolerable in the presence of soft tissue damage. It is important, however, to check for associated spinal sources of symptoms.

The patterns of pain from facet dysfunction do not seem to follow dermatome or myotome distribution and can be very variable. While certain distributions of pain are suggestive and localised tenderness is helpful in making a diagnosis, the clinician must bear in mind that, as Fred Mitchell Jr (DO) has often remarked, 'pain is a liar'. The key criterion is blocked movement. The absence of localised pain does not rule out a problem, nor does it eliminate the lesion as a source of distal pain. With experience comes clinical acumen and, with this, the possible sources of persistent pain become less confusing. Common sense dictates the management of such problems; one cannot diagnose joint dysfunction in the presence of contused tissue. Once the soft tissue injury has healed the assessment of joint mobility is tolerable to the patient. If there is residual pain in situations where the tissue damage is considered to have healed, or the fracture has healed, the source of pain may well be joint dysfunction.

There is one aspect of trauma which can have severe consequences if the surgeon is not aware of the possibility of a concurrent spinal joint lesion. That is pain and stiffness followed by puffy moist hyperaesthetic tissue and bone demineralisation, known as Sudeck's atrophy or the Sudeck–Leriche syndrome. Often the injury is minor or trivial. The shoulder–hand syndrome is probably the result of a similar phenomenon. Causalgia, as in Mitchell's classical description in nerve injuries during the American Civil War, may well be part of the same process. The injury may have been trivial but the burning, incapacitating pain so easily triggered and accompanied by smooth glossy skin, wet with sweat, is far from trivial for the patient. Although sympathectomy has been found to be effective in some cases, the role of the upper thoracic and even the cervical spine in generating sympathetic vasomotor changes has not been recognised. In these cases there is always dysfunction in the upper thoracic or cervical joints and treatment of this is not invasive. When given early, this treatment is usually very effective but, unfortunately, if the syndrome is fully developed, the results are less good. This is a good reason for screening the upper spine in every patient who shows any signs that suggest the possible start of this complication.

In the practice of one of the authors, very many wrist fractures were seen and treated. It became a routine to examine the upper spine of every patient who, after 3 or 4 days, had persistent pain, swelling of the digits or otherwise unexplained stiffness. These cases were common and responded rapidly to treatment of the spinal joint dysfunction that was invariably present. Often only one treatment was required. During the ensuing period of about 10 years the only case of sympathetic dystrophy seen in the practice was one who had had the first 6 weeks treatment at the 'Royal Elsewhere Infirmary'.

In very few such cases is there any complaint of back or neck pain. The diagnosis is made by finding restriction of movement and tissue tension abnormality when one takes the trouble to examine the spine.

The authors are well aware of the disbelief with which some physicians will read this section. Unless some better approach is known, it is recommended that this approach should be tried and the results observed.

WHIPLASH

The injury that acquires the label of 'whiplash' seems usually to be precipitated by a rear-end motor vehicle collision. Pain is generally manifest some hours after the accident but severe distress is often not in evidence until the following day. Whiplash is usually considered to be restricted to the neck, but involvement of the lumbosacral area is common, and indeed the injuries can be widespread. The other areas are overlooked often because the symptoms are minor in comparison to the distress generated by the neck injury.

It is unlikely that joint dysfunction can be diagnosed specifically in the early stages; the acute tissue injury makes it impossible to palpate joint mobility, and specific examination is not tolerated. Early manual treatment, however, does have a place; indirect manipulation can greatly shorten the course of recovery. Relief of pain can be achieved by putting the joint and associated soft tissues at their position of greatest ease. This helps to halt inappropriate proprioceptive activity. This position is held for perhaps a minute and a half and then the neck is very slowly returned to the neutral position. Contused tissues are likely to be healed in about 6 weeks after the accident. At this stage, isometric mobilisation can be instituted, depending on tolerance to palpation and the specific diagnosis of joint dysfunction. The upper thoracic spine is very commonly involved, as is the upper cervical.

It is worth repeating that is is advisable to restrict manipulation of the upper cervical spine to muscle energy techniques. The well-documented occlusion of the vertebral artery is associated with a position of hyperextension and rotation. The course of this artery as it enters the cranial cavity through the foramen magnum makes it vulnerable at that level. Regardless of the type of manipulation used, the risk of a severe vascular complication remains, although small. It was thought formerly that a position of slight flexion would ensure safety, but the consensus now is that direct thrust manipulation should not be used in the upper cervical spine. Isometric manipulation or muscle energy is gentle, tolerable and most unlikely to cause trouble. It is the recommended approach to the upper cervical spine, and the only method described in this book.

Occipital headache radiating anteriorly over the skull to the retro-orbital areas is an almost invariable aspect of whiplash. Sometimes there are complaints of visual disturbances such as difficulty in focusing and there may be tinnitus. Pain in the maxilla or mandible may suggest temporomandibular joint dysfunction, and, in fact, this may be present as an additional factor. There must be careful examination for C1–2 or C2–3 restriction, but relief of symptoms by treating the cervical lesions alone is not certain. There appears to be a cranial component for which 'occipital decompression' may be helpful, and temporal bone restrictions can also be significant. Osteopathic craniosacral theory is outside the scope of this book but can be important in the treatment of whiplash, and readers are referred to works on the subject. [2,3]

The sacroiliac joints are also important whether they are considered as part of the craniosacral mechanism or as structures involved in the injury. The evidence strongly suggests that the mechanism of injury in rear-end collisions is not the simple hyperextension that at one time it was thought to be. The slope of the seat is such that there is often enough upward force on the body to cause the head to strike the roof and in very many instances there is evidence of disturbance of pelvic function as well.

ORGANIC DISEASE

In the presence of systemic disease there is often co-existent somatic dysfunction and it is necessary to evaluate what the contribution of this dysfunction may be to the overall clinical picture. Pain is always debilitating and it can do much for the patient if the stress produced by the pain can be reduced. If it is decided to use manual techniques, the type of manipulation must be selected in reference to the systemic disorder. For instance, thrusting manipulation is traumatic to a small degree, even when performed well, and is contraindicated in the presence of inflammatory joint disease. Muscle energy techniques, however, can be very helpful, although it must be recognised that they are *not* the treatment for rheumatoid arthritis but rather for the superimposed or concurrent joint dysfunction. One of the authors has treated at least two cases with positive tissue typing and symptoms suggestive of Marie–Strümpell spondylitis. The rheumatologist had expressly forbidden manipulative treatment. This would be correct if only thrusting procedures were known. Muscle energy, however, is not contraindicated in the circumstances and, in these two cases, provided rapid relief of the symptoms, indicating that sacroiliitis was not the correct diagnosis. The x-rays were negative.

The idea that organic disease can precipitate musculoskeletal manifestations such as muscle spasm and autonomic reflex activity is well recognised. In contrast, the idea that musculoskeletal dysfunction may precipitate organic problems is usually considered as nothing less than quackery. It is difficult for a traditionally trained physician to accept such a possibility. The thought of treating coronary vascular disease by manipulation seems outrageous, but it should not be rejected out of hand. If autonomic reflex activity is accepted as a vehicle for many of the manifestations of joint or somatic dysfunction, then one can postulate that coronary vasospasm might be a result of somatic dysfunction and, if so, that it might respond to manual management.

One of the authors (JFB) has experience in a case which gives one pause to reflect. A cousin visiting from abroad remarked that since his previous visit he had developed angina. ECG changes were present, and walking for some 180 metres (200 yards) up a slope of 1 in 7 made him need nitroglycerin. Inquiry revealed that he had a history of neck pain and stiffness, although at the time he had no neck symptoms. It was proposed that he should be examined and treated on the basis that any dysfunction found would be treated and the effect on cardiac function observed, if any. Examination did indeed reveal dysfunction in both neck and upper thoracic spine, and treatment on five visits over a 2-week period made a significant difference to the objective signs of joint dysfunction. The effect on cardiac function, or presumably on cardiac function, was remarkable. By the time he was due to return home, he was able to play a full set of tennis followed by a swim with no need of medication. This case does not signify anything other than that an explanation is necessary. The results may not have anything to do with manipulation, but similar observations have been recorded by other practitioners of manual medicine. The cardiac nerve is said to arise from the T_1 to T_4 segments. It has long been speculated that the visceral effects of manipulation are mediated through the autonomic system and vasospasm as a result of autonomic reflex changes is certainly possible. It seems that following up this anecdotal experience is likely to be worth while; only the fool dismisses what he does not understand!

Dr Carl Cook's autobiography *You Must Become A Doctor*[7] contains many references to osteopathic treatment of conditions which we allopathic physicians would consider unresponsive to such measures. The shrunken pathetic little girl with severe asthma, the heavily braced 9-year-old Argentinian boy with only partial control of his legs due to polio, and the man on his death bed from pneumonia superimposed on spinal cord haemorrhage do not seem likely subjects to benefit from manipulation. It would be unreasonable to think that Dr Cook was treating the systemic problems from which these people were suffering, but it is possible that he could make the patients' lot easier by correcting associated spinal or rib cage dysfunction and improve their chances of recovering from conditions for which there was little else to offer. Bronchodilator drugs are an essential part of the modern treatment for asthma and emphysema. So far as we know, their effects are mediated through the parasympathetic system. It is also through the autonomic system that manipulation is thought to have its visceral effects, and the concept that it might help to reduce smooth muscle spasm is not contrary to basic physiology.

There is a complicating factor in this. The remarkably rapid feeling of well-being experienced after successful treatment suggests that manipulation releases endorphins. In this respect it would be similar to exercise. This may explain why some patients see the need for the frequent treatment which is practised and encouraged by certain groups. If the joints needing treatment are not identified and the restriction to movement not resolved, the benefit from manipulative treatment is likely to be brief. Repetitive treatment over a long term indicates failure to diagnose correctly, failure to give satisfactory treatment, or that there is some factor present other than simple joint dysfunction. There are patients in whom the primary condition cannot be relieved but for whom manipulation may make life easier; in such cases, continuing treatment over long periods may be justified but the reasons for this should be clearly understood by both manipulator and patient.

EXERCISE AND POSTURE

Advice on posture, how to stand, how to sit, on sleeping positions and sleeping surfaces, on pillows and on what to do and what not to do is proffered at length by physicians and therapists alike. There is a plethora of advice on exercise, much of it conflicting and much of it without either scientific foundation or evidence that the individual who adheres rigidly to the programme will be any better off. There does not seem to be a correct way of lifting. The concept behind trunk flexion exercises is that weak abdominal muscles and poor posture are important in the generation of joint dysfunction and hence back pain. This is probably valid for the sedentary individual but it remains theory and is sometimes carried to absurd lengths as, for instance, in the experience of one of the authors (EAD), when athletes in top physical shape had been berated for not putting enough effort into their trunk flexion exercises to control their back pain! Trunk flexion exercises can compensate to some extent for joint dysfunction and thereby help some patients, but other practitioners advocate extension exercises and these too can be helpful to some patients. Their opponents' argument that they have never seen weak back muscles is clearly invalid.

Exercises have been the standard management of back pain for decades. They cannot, however, be universally applied; some exercises will precipitate pain in some patients and relief in others. The advice to avoid such activities as jogging ignores the claims that devotees of this exercise in general feel relief of back pain. Avoiding shovelling or lifting because it precipitates back pain is common sense; in our experience, the joint blockage or dysfunction which causes the pain is not going to resolve spontaneously. Even if it subsides with rest, resumption of physical activity will be likely to cause a recurrence of symptoms.

The economic implications of inadequate treatment of joint dysfunction are formidable, particularly for those who earn their living by physical labour. Statistics from one of the Workers Compensation Boards indicate that fewer than 2% of individuals who have been unable to return to work for a 2-year period, because of back pain, are ever likely to do so. That what is so often a simple and correctable, mechanical problem should cause such distress is appalling.

Only the ability to resume all normal activity indicates fully successful treatment. The necessity of avoiding certain physical acts suggests less than full recovery. Certain individuals do appear to be prone to recurrent lesions, for whatever reason, and in these an occupational review would seem warranted. People engaged in physical labour are probably more at risk of recurrence through excess leverage, unguarded movement or unphysiological posture but it ought to be possible to control these episodes by correct treatment. Exercise must be regarded as an adjunct to treatment rather than the definitive management.

PREVENTIVE MANIPULATION

Prophylactic manipulation is recommended by Karel Lewit.[8] He points out that certain occupations are particularly subject to joint dysfunction, the athlete is mentioned as the prime example. Chiropractors often recommend and practise preventive manipulation. There is no doubt that some individuals are particularly prone to joint dysfunction and, either because of their physical demands or because of prolonged adoption of certain postures, some occupations do tend to cause recurrent joint problems. Activities such as repeated stooping or lifting are frequently associated with the onset of back pain.

A basic principle of manual medicine is ignored by some of the advocates of preventive manipulation. Manipulation should be carried out only for a specific diagnosis of joint blockage or dysfunction and the idea that manipulation on a regular basis will prevent the development of such lesions has no foundation. Regular examination for joint dysfunction in certain occupations is more defensible, but it is unlikely to be effective because such examination would not prevent the un-guarded movement or other strains which appear to be the cause of so many joint problems.

Claims are made by some that they are 'kept going' by regular manipulation and that without it they are in pain or are unable to remain at work. We suspect that in these cases there is one of three factors: they have become 'addicted' to the feeling generated by endorphin release, the key joint has not been treated, or the joint dysfunction is not the primary problem and further diagnosis is needed.

JOINT CRACKING

The audible snap associated with direct thrust manipulation is thought to be due to the phenomenon of cavitation. The snap sometimes occurs with muscle energy techniques, although these are usually silent. The only significance of the noise is a confirmation that joint distraction has taken place. It does not indicate anything about the joint, nor does it confirm the diagnosis, a normal joint will snap just like one that is restricted. While the sound pleases some patients, it may alarm others. The occurrence of a snap does not prove the success of the treatment or remove the need for re-examination.

REFERENCES

1. Nachemson A. L. (1979). A critical look at the treatment of low back pain. *Scand J. Rehab. Med;* 11:143–147.
2. Magoun H. I. (1976). *Osteopathy in the Cranial Field*, 3rd edn. Kirksville: The Journal Printing Co.
3. Gehin A. (1985). *Atlas of Manipulative Techniques for the Cranium and Face*. Seattle: Eastland Press.
4. Maigne R. (1980). Low back pain of lumbar origin. *Arch. Phys. Med. Rehab;* 61:389–395.
5. Quinet R. J., Hadler N. M. (1979). Diagnosis and treatment of backache. *Seminars in Arthritis and Rheumatism;* 4:271–287.
6. Andersson G. B. (1981). Epidemiologic aspects of low back pain in industry. *Spine;* 6:53–60.
7. Cook C. M. (1982). *You Must Become a Doctor*. Oxford: Oxford University Press.
8. Lewit K. (1985). *Manipulative Therapy in Rehabilitation of the Motor System*. London: Butterworth.

Chapter 15

The Validation of Manipulation

Manipulation in the eyes of the academician remains 'not proven'. No study has been able to show that it is more effective than anything else, at least regarding back pain.[1] In this it shares, with almost every surgical procedure, the lack of proof by randomised, controlled evaluation.[2] The perception, however, is different. Many surgical procedures enjoy the respectability of acceptance because they have been the indicated solution for a considerable period, are carried out by eminent surgeons and are performed in teaching centres. Indeed, one would not think of denying surgical relief for the obvious on the pedantic basis that there is no randomised, controlled trial. As time goes by, statistics are apt to cause questioning and a revision of attitudes.[3] For example, the number of laminectomies and decompressions for presumed herniation of the nucleus pulposus has fallen, not only because of better selection, but also because the statistics indicating a poor outcome have forced a harder look at the procedure. Recent figures suggest that less than 1% of back pain falls into the realm of surgical decompression or chymopapain injection.[4] The latter appears to be falling out of favour because of the low percentage of good results and the incidence of serious complications. Carotid endarterectomy is another example. For years it has been a surgical procedure of considerable risk and high drama, thought to make the difference between a normal life and hemiplegia or worse. It is still considered to be respectable surgery, but only recently has a multicentre study been launched to determine its efficacy.[5] It may well be that carotid endarterectomy will be vindicated by the study but at present, like manipulation, it remains 'not proven'.

Why then is the concept of manipulation seen as less than acceptable? The label of 'unscientific' is not enough to justify the vitriolic attacks aimed at it by otherwise reasonable physicians. There are ample historical reasons for doubt about manual medicine, but the startling successes which have been noted do not deserve to be dismissed as 'the laying on of hands'. It is sad that, at least in English speaking countries, manual medicine has been excluded from the teaching centres. It is as if the institutions that are responsible for research and the advancement of medical science have, in effect, lifted their gowns to avoid contamination with this unseemly practice. It is not easy to formulate a randomised controlled trial in the face of so many variables without the help of those institutions which supposedly exist to teach and to do research. One rarely sees articles in medical journals concerning manual therapy; a comment in one of the manual medicine newsletters suggests that proffered articles drop into the 'deep dark pool of silence'.

The interest of one of the authors in manipulation was kindled by a

growing frustration in treating thoracic pain of apparently musculoskeletal origin. Heat modalities, physical routines such as traction and
exercise seemed to be reasonably effective for cervical and lumbar problems; at least the symptoms abated! The need for a continuous exercise
regime and the avoidance of certain postures and activities, in order to
remain free from pain, could be rationalised. Thoracic pain, however,
persisted regardless of treatment. Some of these patients went to
chiropractors and obtained relief. They would often say 'I went from
doctor to doctor until finally in desperation I went to a chiropractor
and for the first time obtained relief'. The cynic might explain that in
any number of ways, but the message was clear: the chiropractor was
achieving something that the author was not. It has been osteopathic
medicine that has brought enlightenment. Osteopathic theory concerning barriers to joint movement appeals to one exposed to engineering
as well as to medicine; mechanical interference between two moving
surfaces is a simple explanation without any mumbo-jumbo. Pathological tissue is not a factor as far as we know. Unfortunately, there is a
tendency for manual medicine to attract people interested in the meta-
physical, so that initial exposure to some manual practitioners may well
result in disbelief if not consternation.

The public's demand for manipulation is considerable. As far as the
authors are aware, there is no other way to obtain lasting relief for some
of the common musculoskeletal problems and pain syndromes. It is a
service which has not been generally provided by the allopathic medical
profession. In Canada the American-trained DO still cannot obtain a
licence to practise comparable to that of the MD. In Europe the same
is true, and the picture is complicated by the presence of graduates of
colleges which grant the DO degree without the full training in medicine
and surgery given by the American colleges. The field has been left wide
open to the chiropractors and many patients discover that they can provide better relief for certain problems. The medical profession cannot
escape the fact that many chiropractors enjoy thriving practices. The
authors do not endorse chiropractic; we do not agree with some of their
tenets and there is much in the practice of some chiropractors that we
find profoundly disturbing. Unfortunately, in the face of medical disap-
proval, it is often only the chiropractor to whom the public can turn
if they require manipulative treatment. Medicine is failing adequately
to address the common mechanical problems responsible for huge
economic loss in time away from work, disabled workmen, futile medical investigations and in some cases erroneous surgical intervention, to
say nothing of the pain and suffering which is supposed to abate with
time.

Medical practice has drifted steadily into a pool of serological investigation and decisions are often made solely on the results of laboratory
tests. It is disturbing that a decision to operate may be based on a positive
CAT scan, ignoring the 30% false positive rate reported in some studies.[4]
The superb clinical descriptions of early medicine no longer seem
appropriate because the conditions have become rare, but tabes dorsalis,
for example, would probably present a challenge to a recent medical

graduate. The world of enzymes, serum levels, sophisticated vascular studies, radiographic investigation, computerised tomograms, magnetic resonance imaging and ultrasound has pushed aside basic clinical examination and even basic exposure to anatomy. A description approaching 'a sharp nose, hollow eyes, collapsed temples; the ears cold, contracted and their lobes turned out; the skin about the forehead being rough, distended and parched; the colour of the whole face being green, black, livid or lead coloured'[6] is unlikely to be seen in a problem-oriented medical record of today.

Rheumatology, despite its extensive reliance on laboratory investigations and specific radiological signs, remains a clinical specialty; the diagnosis of rheumatoid arthritis is still a clinical one. Like most medical fields, rheumatology continues to strive for specific findings which will make the diagnosis firm and less reliant on the vagaries of clinical observation. The great rheumatologists, however, are still clinicians.

Manual medicine, too, suffers from the longing for something which will place less reliance on the long period of training for tactile sensitivity, a short cut to that elusive ability in palpatory diagnosis which some never seem to achieve.

Some manual practitioners rely on x-rays to determine the problem, this is especially true of certain chiropractors. In the authors' opinion, the precise position of the barrier to joint movement can only be found by sensitive palpation. Manual medicine remains the last purely clinical frontier. The hands of the practitioner of manual medicine may be short and squat with the thick strong fingers of the peasant, or beautiful and slender with the long tapered fingers of the aristocrat, but in common will be sensitivity of varying degree depending on training and genetic gift. Hands are the only tools in this field.

The barrier concept of joint dysfunction is simple; the lesion can be palpated, the remedy is almost instantaneous, of very low risk and very cheap. There is no laboratory study or x-ray investigation that will help in making the diagnosis. The expense lies in the long tedious path of the training of hands to achieve effective tactile skill. It is something that takes perserverance and is not quickly learned. Some individuals are more gifted for tactile perception than others, some may not be able to acquire the skills to manipulate successfully. More important is that there will never be many physicians manipulating as long as manual medicine is excluded from the teaching centres. If the present position continues it may well be that manual medicine will be doomed to be practised by unorthodox schools and probably in a manner which will cause it to be rejected by the medical profession at large.

Manual medicine does need validation in a randomised, controlled trial that would meet the skepticism of its critics. Despite the variables, and there are many, it should not be impossible to establish a valid study. That such a study would only reflect the level of skill of the particular practitioner involved is not significant as long as he possesses a high degree of skill and experience. The unfortunate fact, however, is that the results would not be reproducible by anyone without manual medicine skills. One suspects that no notice would be taken even if such an investigation were found to be successful.

There is a duty, however, to explain and to justify and to convince the slow-reacting medical profession that it cannot continue to deny to its graduates this tool of incalculable value. The ground rules for a study must be laid out with care.

1. There must be a diagnosis. To study non-specific back pain would be like studying a fracture with the location unspecified. The point is made in this book that it is essential to localise the barrier in all three planes before one can talk about a specific diagnosis.

2. The necessity of looking at other levels must be allowed for. Treatment of one joint alone will usually not be fully successful because of the interplay of dysfunctions on each other even at a distance. For example, the symptom of headache may be directly related to a disturbance of motion in a cervical segment but the primary dysfunction may even be sacroiliac.

3. The assessment of results presents serious difficulties. For instance, traditional application of heat and exercise will often result in a lessening of symptoms. This may also happen with rest and the passage of time. How does one distinguish these effects from those of treatment by manipulation? Many attempts have been made to quantify pain but none of these yet seems good enough to be relied on for measurement of results of this nature. A well-devised functional evaluation should be more productive. Many patients treated by physiotherapists, in particular, end up with warnings as to what they must do and what they must not do, and with exercise programmes which depend more on the particular practitioner than on the problem being treated. Ability to return to work and to carry on normal daily activity without restriction is a much more stringent test and is likely to be valuable in making an assessment. A functional evaluation using specified tasks would be helpful if allowance were made for the state of general physical fitness of the subject. Athletes, who have a high incidence of spinal joint dysfunction, are likely to outperform unfit, sedentary workers in any functional evaluation, even when the former have dysfunctions and the latter have not. Another difficulty is in the probability that some of those in the investigation will, before the assessment, have had a further strain to their spinal joints because these are so common.

An alternative means of measuring the success of treatment would be by the rate of return to work of injured workers. Compensation Board statistics indicate that individuals with back injuries who have not returned to work within 2 years of their accidents are unlikely ever to do so. The rate of return is of the order of 1% or 2%. Even a small increase in this percentage would be significant, but the factors that militate against a satisfactory outcome in a group such as this are formidable. Any workers compensation group is tainted by the spectre of secondary gain and by the psychological devastation of a long period of unemployment. These very factors would reflect startlingly well on a satisfactory outcome, should one have the courage to conduct such a study.

The outcome of manipulative treatment depends on many factors, chief among which is the skill of the treating practitioner. He or she must be able to detect and define the lesion using subtle clinical findings and must be able to pinpoint the barrier to joint movement. The more closely the barrier is engaged, the easier and gentler the treatment becomes. A tense and guarded patient can make attempted diagnosis a futile exercise. One cannot palpate subtle losses in joint movement in the face of rigidly held muscles. Gaining the patient's confidence is paramount, but occasionally it will not be forthcoming. Some people do not like to be touched, turned or twisted and it is better not to attempt this very physical treatment in such circumstances. Even if the diagnosis can be made, attempts to treat would be futile.

In most cases the symptoms appear to abate with time. Usually there is a tendency for recurrence, precipitated by physical activity or certain postures, or anything which will decompensate the mechanical lesion. In our experience they do not often resolve spontaneously.

To map out an effective randomised controlled study is not an easy matter. Another inconclusive study added to those already done would not be helpful. This could easily happen, even if some of the shortcomings of the previous studies can be seen. None of those perused says enough about the skill of the manipulator. Nor is there adequate specificity in defining the lesion treated. The concept that useful information could be obtained from a study of 'rotational manipulation of the spine for non-specific back pain' is completely at variance with the authors' idea of how manipulative treatment ought to be performed.

REFERENCES

1. Buerger A., Greenman P. E. (1985). *Empirical Approaches to the Validation of Spinal Manipulation*. Springfield, Ill: Charles C Thomas.
2. Editorial (1986). The epistemology of surgery. *Lancet*; 1:656–657.
3. Nachemson A. L. (1979). A critical look at the treatment of low back pain. *Scand. J. Rehab. Med*; 11:143–147.
4. Hudgins W. (1983). Computer-aided diagnosis in lumbar disc herniation. *Spine*; 8:604–615.
5. Lechky O. (1986). Carotid endarterectomy goes on trial. *Medical Post*; 22, No. 5. Toronto.
6. Adams F. (1886). *The Genuine Works of Hippocrates*. New York: Wood.

Index